T0075020

Health Informatics

Sajeesh Kumar • Helen Snooks
(Editors)

Kathryn J. Hannah • Marion J. Ball
(Series Editors)

Telenursing

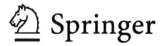 Springer

Editors
Sajeesh Kumar, PhD
Department of Health information
Management
School of Health and Rehabilitation
Sciences
University of Pittsburgh
Pittsburgh, Pennsylvania
USA

Helen Sneeks
Centre for Health, Information, Research
and Evaluation (CHIRAL)
Swansea University
Swansea, Cardiff
UK

ISBN 978-0-85729-528-6   e-ISBN 978-0-85729-529-3
DOI 10.1007/978-0-85729-529-3
Springer London Dordrecht Heidelberg New York

British Library Cataloguing in Publication Data
A catalogue record for this book is available from the British Library

Library of Congress Control Number: 2011928410

© Springer-Verlag London Limited 2011
Apart from any fair dealing for the purposes of research or private study, or criticism or review, as permitted under the Copyright, Designs and Patents Act 1988, this publication may only be reproduced, stored or transmitted, in any form or by any means, with the prior permission in writing of the publishers, or in the case of reprographic reproduction in accordance with the terms of licenses issued by the Copyright Licensing Agency. Enquiries concerning reproduction outside those terms should be sent to the publishers.
The use of registered names, trademarks, etc., in this publication does not imply, even in the absence of a specific statement, that such names are exempt from the relevant laws and regulations and therefore free for general use.
Product liability: The publisher can give no guarantee for information about drug dosage and application thereof contained in this book. In every individual case the respective user must check its accuracy by consulting other pharmaceutical literature.

Cover design: eStudioCalamar, Figueres/Berlin

Printed on acid-free paper

Springer is part of Springer Science+Business Media (www.springer.com)

Series Preface

This series is directed to healthcare professionals leading the transformation of healthcare by using information and knowledge. For over 20 years, Health Informatics has offered a broad range of titles: some address specific professions such as nursing, medicine, and health administration; others cover special areas of practice such as trauma and radiology; still other books in the series focus on interdisciplinary issues, such as the computer based patient record, electronic health records, and networked healthcare systems. Editors and authors, eminent experts in their fields, offer their accounts of innovations in health informatics. Increasingly, these accounts go beyond hardware and software to address the role of information in influencing the transformation of healthcare delivery systems around the world. The series also increasingly focuses on the users of the information and systems: the organizational, behavioral, and societal changes that accompany the diffusion of information technology in health services environments.

Developments in healthcare delivery are constant; in recent years, bioinformatics has emerged as a new field in health informatics to support emerging and ongoing developments in molecular biology. At the same time, further evolution of the field of health informatics is reflected in the introduction of concepts at the macro or health systems delivery level with major national initiatives related to electronic health records (EHR), data standards, and public health informatics.

These changes will continue to shape health services in the twenty-first century. By making full and creative use of the technology to tame data and to transform information, Health Informatics will foster the development and use of new knowledge in healthcare.

Kathryn J. Hannah
Marion J. Ball

Preface

Developments in telenursing are progressing at a great speed. As a consequence, there is a need for a broad overview of the field. This first ever book on telenursing is presented in such a way that it should make it accessible to anyone, independent of their knowledge of technology. The text is designed to be used by *all* professionals, including nurses, physicians, all allied health professionals and computer scientists.

In a very short time, driven by technical developments, the field of telenursing has become too extensive to be covered by only a small number of experts. Therefore, this *Telenursing* book has been written with chapter contributions from a host of renowned international authorities in telenursing (see the Table of Contents and the List of Contributors). This ensures that the subject matter focusing on recent advances in telenursing is truly up to date. Our guiding hope during this task was that as editors of multiple chapters we could still write with a single voice and keep the content coherent and simple. We hope that the clarity of this book makes up for any limitations in its comprehensiveness.

The editors took much care that this *Telenursing* book would not become merely a collection of separate chapters but, rather, would offer a consistent and structured overview of the field. We are aware that there is still considerable room for improvement and that certain elements of telenursing are not fully covered, such as legal and reimbursement policies. The editors invite readers to forward their valuable comments and feedback to further improve and expand future editions of this *Telenursing* book.

Books on theoretical and technical aspects inevitably use technical jargon, and this book is no exception. Although jargon is minimised, it cannot be eliminated without retreating to a more superficial level of coverage. The reader's understanding of the jargon will vary based on their backgrounds, but anyone with some background in computers, nursing and/or health would be able to understand most of the terms used. In any case, an attempt has been made to define all jargon terms in the Glossary.

This *Telenursing book* has been organised systematically. The format and length of each chapter are standardised, thus ensuring that the content is concise and easy to read. Every chapter provides a comprehensive list of citations and references for further reading. Figure drawings and clinical photographs throughout the book illustrate and illuminate the text well, providing its readers with high-quality visual reference material. Particularly useful features of this text are that each chapter has a summary of salient points for the reader.

The book consists of 17 chapters and begins with a brief introductory chapter explaining the basic concepts that are mainstay to telenursing, and subsequent chapters are built upon those foundations, through the experiences from various nations. Within each chapter, the goal is to provide a comprehensive overview of the topic. The final chapter covers future directions of telenursing.

This book would not have been possible without the contribution from various people. We acknowledge and appreciate the assistance of all reviewers and Ms. Latika Hans, editorial assistant from Bangalore, India. We would like to thank all authors for making this book possible through their contributions and constant support.

Sajeesh Kumar
Helen Snooks

Contents

Contributors

Leila Maria Marchi Alves
University of São Paulo, Ribeirão Preto
College of Nursing,
Ribeirão Preto, Brazil/São Paulo, Brazil

Antonia Arnaert
School of Nursing, McGill University,
Montreal, QC, Canada

Masumi Azuma
Graduate School of Applied Informatics,
University of Hyogo,
Kobe, Hyogo, Japan

Susan Bell
Choose Independence, Peterborough, UK

Simone De Godoy
University of São Paulo, Ribeirão Preto
College of Nursing, Ribeirão Preto,
Brazil/São Paulo, Brazil

I. Ellis
La Trobe Rural Health School, Bendigo,
VIC, Australia

Jill Fortuin
Telemedicine Platform, Medical Research
Council, Cape Town, South Africa

Kazimierz Frączkowski
Institute of Informatics, Wroclaw
University of Technology, Wroclaw,
Poland

K. Ganapathy
Apollo Telemedicine Networking
Foundation, Apollo Hospitals, Chennai,
TN, India

Francisco Gonzalez
Department of Physiology, School of
Medicine, Santiago de Compostela, Spain
Service of Ophthalmology, Complejo
Hospitalario Universitario de Santiago de
Compostela, Santiago de Compostela,
Spain

Janet L. Grady
Nursing Program at UPJ,
University of Pittsburgh at Johnstown,
Johnstown, PA, USA

Janet Harp
Medibank Health Solutions NZ Ltd,
Wellington, New Zealand

G. Hercelinskyj
La Trobe Rural Health School, Bendigo,
VIC, Australia

Inger Holmström
Department of Public Health and Caring
Sciences, Uppsala University, Health
Services Research, Uppsala, Sweden

Takayasu Kawaguchi
Doctoral Program in Nursing Sciences,
Graduate School of Comprehensive
Human Sciences, University of Tsukuba,
Tsukuba, Ibaraki, Japan

Sajeesh Kumar
Department of Health Information
Management, School of Health &
Rehabilitation Sciences, University of
Pittsburgh, Pittsburgh, PA, USA

Fiona Macfarlane
School of Nursing, McGill University,
Westmount, QC, Canada

Alessandra Mazzo
University of São Paulo, Ribeirão Preto
College of Nursing, Ribeirão Preto,
Brazil/São Paulo, Brazil

B. McEwan
La Trobe Rural Health School, Bendigo,
VIC, Australia

Isabel Amélia Costa Mendes
University of São Paulo, Ribeirão Preto
College of Nursing, Ribeirão Preto,
Brazil/São Paulo, Brazil

Joselito M. Montalban
University of the Philippines in Manila,
Cagayan de Oro, Philippines

Emilio Morete
Service of Neumology, Complejo
Hospitalario Universitario de Santiago de
Compostela, Santiago de Compostela,
Spain

Maria Suely Nogueira
University of São Paulo, Ribeirão Preto
College of Nursing, Ribeirão Preto,
Brazil/São Paulo, Brazil

Hyeoun-Ae Park
College of Nursing, Seoul National
University, Chongno-gu, Seoul, South
Korea

Julie Peconi
Centre for Health Information Research and
Evaluation (CHIRAL), College of Medicine,
Swansea University, Swansea, UK

Alison Porter
Centre for Health Information Research
and Evaluation (CHIRAL), School of
Medicine, Swansea University, Swansea,
UK

Elaine Maria Leite Rangel
Health Sciences Center, Department of
Nursing, Federal University of Piauí,
Teresina, Brazil/Piauí, Brazil

Aditi Ravindra
Apollo Telemedicine Networking
Foundation, Apollo Hospitals, Chennai,
TN, India

Masae Satoh
Division of Nursing Sciences, Faculty of
Health Sciences, Tokyo Metropolitan
University, Arakawa-ku, Tokyo, Japan

Ann Saxon
Continuing Development Division,
School of Health, University of
Wolverhampton, Walsall, UK

Carlos Alberto Seixas
University of São Paulo, Ribeirão Preto
College of Nursing, Ribeirão Preto,
Brazil/São Paulo, Brazil

Helen Snooks
Centre for Health Information Research
and Evaluation (CHIRAL), School of
Medicine, Swansea University, Swansea,
UK

Ian St George
Medibank Health Solutions NZ Ltd,
Wellington, New Zealand

Maria Auxiliadora Trevizan
University of São Paulo,
Ribeirão Preto College of Nursing,
Ribeirão Preto, Brazil/São Paulo,
Brazil

Sinclair Wynchank
Telemedicine Platform,
Medical Research Council,
Cape Town, South Africa

Yoji Yoshioka
Doctoral Program in Nursing Sciences,
Graduate School of Comprehensive
Human Sciencess, University of Tsukuba,
Tsukuba, Ibaraki, Japan

Eun Kyoung Yun
College of Nursing Science, Kyung Hee
University, Dongdaemun-gu, Seoul,
South Korea

Carlos Zamarrón
Service of Neumology, Complejo
Hospitalario Universitario de Santiago de
Compostela, Santiago de Compostela,
Spain

Antoni Zwiefka
The Marshal's Office of Lower Silesia,
Wroclaw, Poland

Introduction to Telenursing

1

Sajeesh Kumar

1.1
Introduction to Telemedicine

Telemedicine is a method by which patients can be examined, investigated, monitored, and treated, with the patient and the doctor being located at different places. Tele is a Greek word meaning "distance," and Mederi is a Latin word meaning "to heal." Although initially considered "futuristic" and "experimental," telemedicine is today a reality and has come to stay. In telemedicine one transfers the expertise, not the patient. Hospitals of the future will drain patients from all over the world without geographical limitations. High-quality medical services can be brought to the patient, rather than transporting the patient to distant and expensive tertiary-care centers. A major goal of telemedicine is to eliminate unnecessary traveling of patients and their escorts. Image acquisition, image storage, image display and processing, and image transfer represent the basis of telemedicine. Telemedicine is becoming an integral part of health-care services in several countries.

1.2
What Is Telenursing?

Telenursing is the use of telecommunications and information technology to provide nursing practice at a distance. This can be something as simple as faxing medical records to the more complex delivery of nursing care to patients' home through the use of cameras and computer technologies.

S. Kumar
Department of Health Information Management, School of Health & Rehabilitation Sciences, University of Pittsburgh, 6022 Forbes Tower, 15260 Pittsburgh, PA, USA
e-mail: sajeeshkr@yahoo.com

S. Kumar and H. Snooks (eds.), *Telenursing*, Health Informatics,
DOI: 10.1007/978-0-85729-529-3_1, © Springer-Verlag London Limited 2011

1.3
Scope of Telenursing

Telenursing is growing at a faster rate in many countries due to several factors: the preoccupation in driving down the costs of health care, an increase in the number of aging and chronically ill population, and the increase in coverage of health care to distant, rural, small, or sparsely populated regions. Among its many benefits, telenursing may help solve increasing shortages of nurses, reduce distances and save travel time, and keep patients out of hospital.

The most common use of telenursing is by call centers operated by managed care organizations, which are staffed by registered nurses who act as case managers or perform patient triage, information and counseling as a means of regulating patient access and flow and decreasing the use of emergency rooms.

Telenursing has also been used as a tool in home nursing. For example, patients who are immobilized or live in remote or difficult-to-reach places, or citizens who have chronic ailments, such as chronic obstructive pulmonary disease or diabetes, or disabilitating diseases, such as neural degenerative diseases (Parkinson's disease, Alzheimer's disease), may stay at home and be "visited" and assisted regularly by a nurse via videoconferencing, Internet, videophone, etc. Still other applications of home care are the care of patients in immediate post-surgical situations, and the care of wounds, ostomies, handicapped individuals, etc.[4,6-8]

Telenursing can also provide opportunities for patient education, nursing teleconsultations, examination of results of medical tests and examinations, and assistance to physicians in the implementation of medical treatment protocols.[1,2]

Potential applications of telenursing may also include[3,9]

- Training nurses remotely.
- Assisting and training nurses in developing countries.
- Nursing care for soldiers on or near the battlefield.
- Collaborating and mentoring by nurses around the globe.

1.4
Current Issues

Telenursing is fraught with potential legal, ethical, and regulatory issues, as it happens with telehealth as a whole.[5] In many countries, interstate and intercountry practice of telenursing is forbidden (the attending nurse must have a licence both in his/her state/country of residence and in the state/country where the patient receiving telecare is located). Legal issues such as accountability, malpractice, etc. are also still largely unsolved and difficult to address.

In addition, there are many considerations related to patient confidentiality and safety of clinical data. Civil and criminal penalties can thus be brought against health-care providers if they do not conform to the laws of the state. Telenursing practitioners should take this into consideration, in addition to be ensuring safe and ethical practice with the privacy and confidentiality of patient information.

1.5
Summary

- Telenursing is the use of telecommunications and information technology to provide nursing practice at a distance, which may help solve increasing shortages of nurses, reduce distances and save travel time, and keep patients out of hospital.
- The most common use of telenursing is by call centers staffed by registered nurses who regulate patient access and flow and decrease the use of emergency rooms.
- Telenursing has also been used as a tool in home nursing, where immobilized patients, those living in remote areas or those with chronic ailments may stay at home and be visited and assisted regularly by a nurse via videoconferencing, Internet, videophone, etc.
- Telenursing is fraught with potential legal, ethical, and regulatory issues, as it happens with telehealth as a whole.
- In addition to ensuring safe and ethical practice, telenursing practitioners should also take into consideration the privacy and confidentiality of patient information.

References

1. Cook PF, McCabe MM, Emiliozzi S, et al. Telephone nurse counseling improves HIV medication adherence: an effectiveness study. *J Assoc Nurses AIDS Care*. 2009;20(4):316-325.
2. Dias VP, Witt RR, Silveira DT, et al. Telenursing in primary health care: report of experience in southern Brazil. *Stud Health Technol Inform*. 2009;146:202-206.
3. Flippin C. Military nursing licensure that transcends borders. *Plast Surg Nurs*. 2009;29(3): 149-150.
4. Jensen L, Leeman-Castillo B, Coronel SM, et al. Impact of a nurse telephone intervention among high-cardiovascular-risk, health fair participants. *J Cardiovasc Nurs*. 2009;24(6): 447-453.
5. Litchfield SM. Update on the nurse licensure compact. *AAOHN J*. 2010;58(7):277-279.
6. Lyndon H, Tyas D. Telehealth enhances self care and independence in people with long term conditions. *Nurs Times*. 2010;106(26):12-13.
7. Naditz A. Telenursing: front-line applications of telehealthcare delivery. *Telemed J E Health*. 2009;15(9):825-829.
8. Sherrard H, Struthers C, Kearns SA, et al. Using technology to create a medication safety net for cardiac surgery patients: a nurse-led randomized control trial. *Can J Cardiovasc Nurs*. 2009;19(3):9-15.
9. Terry M, Halstead LS, O'Hare P, et al. Feasibility study of home care wound management using telemedicine. *Adv Skin Wound Care*. 2009;22(8):358-364.

Teaching Telenursing with the Charles Darwin University Virtual Hospital™

2

I. Ellis, G Hercelinskyj, and B. McEwan

Abbreviations

CDU   Charles Darwin University
RFDS   Royal Flying Doctor Service
vHospital™   Charles Darwin University Virtual Hospital™

2.1
Introduction

The American Academy of Ambulatory Care Nursing defines telenursing as "the delivery, management, and coordination of care and services provided via telecommunications technology within the domain of nursing."[1] This ranges from telephone triage, digital imaging for wound management, to electronic discharge planning. Telenursing is not a new field in Australia. In 1912, the Australian Inland Mission established nursing posts where nurses in outback Australia were stationed in remote towns and communities to provide care to the community. This care covered midwifery and the immediate emergency care needs of people suffering from injuries and acute illnesses, and the public health functions of health assessment, immunization, monitoring, and health promotion. By 1929 the Traeger pedal radio was introduced in North Queensland to allow communication between the nursing post and the newly established Royal Flying Doctor Service (RFDS) physician, thereby establishing the first routine telenursing service (Fig. 2.1). Within the first year, the RFDS had made 50 flights and treated 225 people. By 1934 a radio was installed in the aircraft allowing communication to be maintained with the ground. This heralded the first telenursing consultation with the physician in flight from a nurse at the remote town of Innaminka.[8] Today telenursing is widespread. Nursing triage call centers are available in every state and territory in Australia, and nurses routinely communicate with distant specialists using a range of technologies and web-based interfaces such as Wounds West (http://www.health.wa.gov.au/woundswest/home).

I. Ellis (✉)
La Trobe Rural Health School, P.O. Box 199, 3552 Bendigo, Victoria, Australia
e-mail: isabelle.ellis@latrobe.edu.au

S. Kumar and H. Snooks (eds.), *Telenursing*, Health Informatics,
DOI: 10.1007/978-0-85729-529-3_2, © Springer-Verlag London Limited 2011

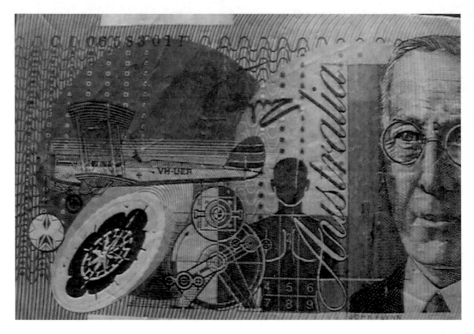

Fig. 2.1 The Australian $20 note has the face of Rev. John Flynn and the pedal radio to his *left*

As nursing educators and academics endeavor to ensure that the teaching and learning environment keeps pace with the clinical environment, there is a need to ensure that students are engaged with current and emerging telenursing technologies as undergraduates. The Charles Darwin University (CDU) Virtual Hospital™ also known as the vHospital™ has been developed to ensure that students are presented with a rich online learning environment that encompasses a range of telenursing activities. This chapter presents an overview of the vHospital, highlighting the way that students experience telenursing through a range of interactive case studies.

2.2
Background

Using case histories is a routine teaching practice in undergraduate health science courses. Case-based learning, problem-based learning, and enquiry-based learning are all methodologies that use cases as their primary learning objects. Some of the cases are based on real patient data and some are developed by the academics to illustrate a range of principles. What cases have in common is that they are chosen for their relevance to the teaching context and the learning objectives of the course of study. The vHospital cases are developed by academics and industry partners to highlight the learning outcomes. They use actual patient data that are brought together with fictional elements to follow patients on their journey from their home environment into the hospital and then on to discharge.

The cases in the vHospital are currently used by CDU in a case-based learning mode. Case-based learning was chosen as the teaching methodology as it facilitates development of professional knowledge and behaviors expected of the beginning practitioner; it enables students to see skills in context rather than a checklist of procedures that must be mastered.[2] The case-based learning environment reinforces the underlying patient-centered philosophy of the Bachelor of Nursing program. It highlights the fundamental principles that nursing care is concerned with the psychosocial, psychological, and physical well-being of the patient contextualized by their place within their family, community, and society. Case-based learning also allows students to work on their own rather than in small groups as is done in both problem-based learning and enquiry-based learning,[3,7] which is particularly pertinent to students studying in external mode. Australia, as a continent, has many different time zones and students studying externally choose this mode as it allows them to study "anytime/anywhere." The cohort of CDU's nursing students consists of approximately 20% internal and 80% external, many of whom are mature-age students living in rural and remote areas who do not have access to other students during the term time. Many of the students study part time to enable them to continue to work to support families. Case-based learning supports flexibility for students.

Nursing is a practice-based profession; however, the key elements that underpin all nursing practice are "problem solving, decision making, and clinical judgment."[10] Undergraduate nurses need to be able to practice these problem-solving skills. Most teaching simulations are designed to do just that. However, it is difficult to provide a way of ensuring that the consequences of decisions are able to be felt by the student in more than the most rudimentary way, even with high fidelity simulation dummies and well-designed scenarios. The vHospital has taken a range of standard case studies that were used in the medical/surgical nursing and mental health nursing undergraduate units and designed them to be able to be delivered in an online interactive case-based learning environment.

2.3
Learning Telewound Care

Telewound care is a growing area of telenursing. The key principles of wound management are taught to all nursing undergraduate students. It is clear that as the variety of wound care products increases it is important to teach principles rather than just practices. Wound management has become a specialized field of nursing; however, there is a need to ensure that specialist care is available for people with complex and chronic wounds. A recent study in the USA reported that less than 0.2% of nurses were wound care certified.[11] The opportunity to seek specialist advice for wound care is enhanced by telehealth technologies, and students becoming familiar with the requirements and the skills will ensure that they are able to refer patients appropriately.

2.3.1
The Patient Journey Begins

Students learning wound care in a clinical environment or with a simulation exercise are very frequently first shown the wound and then the patient, or they meet the patient in the context of the clinical setting where wound care is expected to be provided. In the vHospital, students are introduced to the patient in the context of his/her life and observe the situation that made the person seek health care.

2.3.2
The Case

John Wayne is 55 years old and leads a relatively sedentary lifestyle. John lives in a remote Aboriginal community with his wife and children, and his grandchildren. John is the primary income earner for the family. He works as an environmental program supervisor which is an office-based job.

> During the weekends John likes to go hunting with his grandchildren, but nowadays he mostly drives the "Troupie" [the colloquial name for a four wheel drive passenger vehicle] to the waterhole and gets the fire ready while the young ones go out hunting. In the past few months John has been experiencing unusual thirst, dizziness, occasional blurred vision and an awkward feeling of numbness in his right foot. John presents at the remote area nursing post with a non-painful wound on his foot caused by him stepping on a stone. The wound is not healing. The nurse and the visiting doctor consult with John and advise him that he needs to go to town for further tests and to have his wound managed (*Source*: CDU vHospital).

The students are given a picture of John as a person having fun with his grandchildren as well as a picture of the wound on John's foot.

Students also have links within the vHospital to gain more information. The links include cultural considerations, external resources relevant to the case, and a link to the university library where relevant research papers and texts are held in eReserve.

John is brought from his remote clinic by RFDS to the vHospital.

Providing care for John will involve students gaining an understanding of John's psychosocial, psychological, and physical care needs. From the story they are required to identify the relevant forms that will be needed when they admit John. They should assemble a wound care chart, a blood glucose monitoring chart, a nursing history and assessment chart, a general observation chart, a fluid balance chart, and the integrated progress notes.

2.3.3
Providing Telewound Care

Once John is admitted to the ward, students consider John's wound care needs. They are introduced to the tools of telewound care. They are presented with a digital image of John's wound (Fig. 2.2) and a clinical algorithm or decision tree which includes when to take a digital image (Fig. 2.3).

The use of clinical algorithms based on best practice guidelines is a tool of telenursing, as it standardizes decision making and aids nurses on when and where to refer the patient or their information. In the case of telewound care, an image of the wound is indicated if the patient has a wound healing by secondary intention. This would include any burn wound, ulcer, trauma wound that was not sutured, or any surgical wound healing by

Fig. 2.2 Wound image from the vHospital case John Wayne

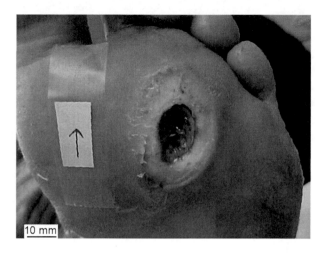

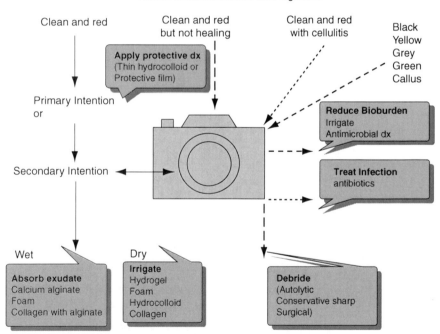

Fig. 2.3 Wound care algorithm from the vHospital case John Wayne

secondary intention. Treatment decisions are based on the algorithm and referral decisions are appropriate to a beginning practitioner, such as the presence of callus requires debridement – refer to wound care nurse consultant.

Once an image is recorded, there is a need to be able to standardize the measurement and assessment of the wound to determine the healing rate. There are a range of tools readily available on the market for wound measurement, including software packages that calibrate and position the images and incorporate the clinical data into one record. It is not the intention to teach the students how to use each or any of these specific tools but to ensure that they can recognize the different types of tissues associated with wounds, such as slough, epithelizing tissue, necrotic tissue, and granular tissue, and can clearly draw around the wound edges and the edges of the various types of tissues. The surface area of the wound is measured and this information becomes part of the clinical notes.

Students have the opportunity to test their skills against an expert. They use an interactive pen tool to draw around the wound; they are then directed to click the link to compare their assessment against that of a wound care nurse consultant. Students are shown a series of clinical photos that indicate that John's wound has healed over time.

John is discharged back to his community before the wound has completely healed. A nursing discharge summary including a wound care electronic discharge summary is provided to the remote area nurse. The final chapter of the John Wayne case involves the remote area nurse requesting a consultation with the vHospital wound care nurse consultant. The image and the information provided show that John's wound has delayed healing and the consultant identifies that there is a buildup of callus on the wound margin; the final student activity requires the student to use the algorithm and provide the correct advice.

2.3.4
Handover

Between each of the chapters of the vHospital cases a handover is provided. This handover is a scripted, recorded handover between one health-care provider and the next, just as would happen at the change of shift or when handing a patient over for theater. The handover is an important communication tool between health-care providers. It is one of the most important patient safety measures in a hospital that takes up approximately 30 min/shift at least three times a day, 365 days/year[9] and is an area that students find difficult to master. In the case of John Wayne there are four handovers: on admission to the ward, between the Aboriginal health worker and the nurse, on discharge back to the community between the ward nurse and the remote area nurse, and a consultation between the remote area nurse and the vHospital wound care nurse consultant; two of these are a telenursing handover. Students need to listen to the handover and record the relevant information. They then use that information to complete the learning activities, such as filling in the clinical observations on the general observation chart or completing the patient history chart.

Remote area nurse to vHospital wound care nurse consultant handover:

Eddie: Hi is Isabelle there?
Isabelle: Speaking
Eddie: Hi Isabelle it Eddie Fielder here, the nurse looking after John Wayne in the community outside of Katherine.
Isabelle: Hi Eddie, I have received the photo you just sent via email. You are doing a fantastic job of healing John's wound.
Eddie: Thanks but the healing rate seems to be slowing now.

Isabelle: Have a look at the wound margin Eddie and tell me what you see?

Eddie: Well I can see that the wound is getting smaller but there appears to be some build up of callus.

Isabelle: Great Eddie. Yes the wound looks really healthy but you will need to debride that callus or the wound won't be able to heal completely. Remember for a wound to heal by secondary intention the epithelial cells need to form a bridge and migrate across the wound one cell at a time and they can't do this if there is callus or a build up of exudate.

Eddie: Thanks Isabelle. Will do. (*Source*: CDU vHospital).

2.3.5
Teaching and Learning Using the vHospital

There are currently six cases in the vHospital. Students access them via the online learning portal of the university, through their relevant subject link. The initial log on screen gives students a video and text introduction, and information on how to navigate their way around the vHospital and how to access additional information and resources. The top right-hand corner of the screen gives a floor plan of the vHospital; as they move their cursor over each of the areas there is a brief description of the clinical setting and the types of procedures that they will be able to see or practice in the area.

Each case is presented as a patient journey, with specific times or events presented as a chapter. In order to move on to the next chapter students are required to complete an activity that forms part of the formative assessment. The activity answers are stored in a database against each student login, and the lecturer is able to see the student's progress by accessing the database for their students.

The cases are designed to incorporate the learning outcomes of the beginning medical surgical nursing unit and the mental health nursing unit. Each of the cases is rich in video and audio learning objects. There are a large number of interactive activities from an interactive stethoscope for hearing breath sounds to interactive forms and interactive procedure setup trolleys. Procedural videos are provided for the nursing procedures and videos have been made to demonstrate the outcomes of the decisions that students make in some of the interactive activities, such as their response to an aggressive patient in the emergency department.

2.3.6
Other Cases in the vHospital

- Peter Abbott is an indigenous member of parliament who finds that he is unable to pass urine; during his hospital journey students prepare him for surgery and follow him through to operation and care for him post-operatively to discharge.
- Judy Thompson is an Australian international aid worker who has recently returned from Thailand and has developed flu-like symptoms. Students are required to triage Judy correctly to avoid starting an outbreak of H1N1 virus. They care for Judy as a medical patient with an acute respiratory illness.

- Beth Sheba crashes her car on the way to work and is brought in by ambulance to the vHospital. Students need to assemble to correct trauma team and care for Beth in the emergency department. She has a head injury and fractured arm. They then follow her through to the ward and provide her with pain management and fracture care.
- Bikey Bob is a tough tattooed biker who presents with chronic diarrhea and pain. Bob requires surgery for ulcerative colitis and students provide him with post-operative abdominal surgical care and stoma care and prepare him for discharge.
- Robert Bogan is a continuation of the Bikey Bob case. Bob is having trouble adjusting to his altered body image now that he has a stoma and develops a mental illness. Students have to manage his aggression in the emergency department so that he can be admitted; then they care for him with his suicide ideation and depression.

2.4
Teaching Clinical Decision Making in the vHospital

Decision making in nursing is complex. Nurses learn to make nursing decisions based on their ability to gather data about a situation, interpret that data, and apply it to a clinical situation as nursing diagnoses and nursing intervention and then monitor the outcome of that decision. It has long been recognized that intelligent computer-based multimedia-simulated decision making can reduce the time to gain practical knowledge. This is readily recognized in pilot and driver training but has rarely been used in nurse training despite being recognized as a useful learning tool.[4,5]

The vHospital contextualizes student learning in real cases. It models good nursing practice and communication and allows students to see the consequences of their decisions played out. Research has reported that students benefit most when the formative feedback from their decision making is available immediately after the decision is made.[5] The vHospital is a safe environment for students to experiment with making a wrong decision. Each of the cases in the vHospital has at least one intelligent-simulated decision-making activity. Each of the clinical decisions has a try-again option, which provides feedback about the consequences of making a different decision. The decisions can be as simple as choosing from five options how long a patient should wait in the emergency department or choosing from three options when to call the doctor based on the patient's Glasgow coma score.

In the case of Judy Thompson, students are given the story that Judy has just returned from working on the Thai–Lao border as a volunteer aid worker in a small village. Judy relates the story of chickens dying in the village. She has returned to Australia and is staying with her sister and her new baby. Judy has developed flu-like symptoms and comes to the vHospital emergency department where she presents at the triage window and gives her video story. Students need to notice that there are a few elements of Judy's story that warrant careful consideration in how they manage Judy's triage category allocation. Knowledge of the triage categories is essential "know what" knowledge and implementing those categories with a patient encounter is "know how" knowledge.[4] The students' decision will impact on Judy's wait in the emergency department waiting area. After choosing a category, students watch a short video clip that resembles security camera footage of the waiting room in fast forward; students see how many people sit next to Judy during her wait and have the potential of contracting Judy's illness. The final video clip is of a news report of Darwin being isolated by air as the result of an outbreak of pandemic flu which was thought to have started in the vHospital (Fig. 2.4).

Intelligent simulation systems are particularly useful in practice-based professions. They offer greater realism than paper-based exercises. Despite the cost of staging and producing the multimedia elements, they are less expensive than role play-based simulations, as the learning object, once created, can be used by many students simultaneously. And if well designed can be used over a number of years. According to Garrett and Callear,[5] intelligent simulations have a "distinct advantage over traditional multimedia systems as they offer the student individualised advice, promoting heuristic learning, rather than generalised didactic instructions" (p. 388).

2.5
Evaluation

There have been several evaluations throughout the development and integration of the Bachelor of Nursing program. Initial evaluation focused on navigation, usability, content relevance, and interest. The participants found the content of the first case (Peter Abbott) engaging and easy to follow but had varied responses to completing the assessment tasks before being allowed to go on to the next chapter. Participants were particularly positive about being able to replay the procedural videos and found the quizzes self-explanatory and the type of feedback useful. The navigation and introduction were changed as a result of this early feedback. More recently, Hercelinskyj and McEwan[6] have reported that learning using the vHospital "helped students to place learning in a context that assisted them to understand the nursing role and responsibilities as well as how nurses work with others in providing patient care." Students reported being able to explore their role as student nurses, in a safe environment, prior to going on clinical placement. The complexities and realities of the nursing role and the importance of communication and teamwork were also areas that students commented on.

2.6
Conclusion

The vHospital is an innovative computer-based learning tool that provides students with an anytime/anywhere media-rich learning environment. The vHospital is designed to be modified and built on over time as cases are built using a template format and then linked into the shell of the vHospital. Telenursing is incorporated as part of the role of the nurse within the vHospital and students are exposed to the tools and processes of telenursing.

Case-based learning is well suited to the development of intelligent simulation, as the cases are designed collaboratively between academics and clinicians to ensure that they

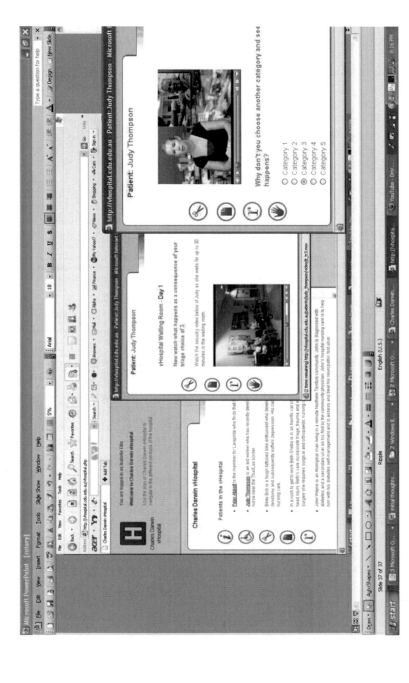

Fig. 2.4 Screen shots from the vHospital case Judy Thompson

are authentic and meet the learning outcomes of the course. Incorporating intelligent simulation activities into the cases acknowledges the complexities of the nursing decision-making process.

2.7
Summary

- Telenursing tools and processes need to be incorporated into nursing education.
- The vHospital™ is a media-rich online case-based learning environment.
- The vHospital™ uses case-based learning as it supports flexibility for students.
- The vHospital™ uses intelligent simulation to teach clinical decision making.

Glossary

Calibrate – To adjust or determine by comparison to a standard.

Case-based learning – Using case studies for learning.

Clinical algorithm – A decision tree to assist with clinical decision making.

Didactic instructions – The delivery of factual information to the student.

Digital imaging – Taking digital photographs.

Enquiry-based learning – A model of teaching that allocates students into groups to work on activities called enquiries.

eReserve – Electronic library holdings.

External mode – A mode of study where students do not meet face-to-face with the lecturer.

Formative assessment – A type of assessment that assesses incremental development of learning.

Heuristic learning – An educational method in which learning takes place through discoveries made through investigations made by the student.

High fidelity simulation dummy – A mannequin that is engineered or designed to model a person as closely as possible.

Interactive pen tool – A drawing tool that is controlled by a computer mouse.

Intelligent simulation – Simulation activities that respond to the student's decisions or choices and allow for alternate choices or decisions to be made.

Learning objects – Elements that are used in teaching; can be physical, audio, video, or a suite of activities.

Learning outcomes – The explicit outcomes that students are required to achieve from a course of study.

Log on screen – The initial Internet screen that the user puts their username and password into to allow access.

Online learning – The delivery of educational materials via the Internet.

Online learning portal – The opening page of an Internet website used for education.

Problem-based learning – A model of teaching that gives students problems to investigate and solve.

Simulation – A method of creating a learning environment or activity that models real life.

Telephone triage – Providing initial assessment of the patient by telephone.

Triage window – A window into the emergency department of a hospital that is manned by a nurse who makes the initial assessment of the patient.

References

1. American Academy of Ambulatory Care Nursing (AAACN). Telehealth, http://www.aaacn.org/cgi-bin/WebObjects/AAACNMain. 2010.
2. Andrew N, McGuinness C, Reid G, Corcoran T. Greater than the sum of its parts: transition into the first year of undergraduate nursing. *Nurse Educ Pract.* 2009;9:13-21.
3. Dochy F, Segers M, Van den Bossche P, Gijbels D. Effects of problem-based learning: a meta-analysis. *Learn Instruct.* 2003;13:533-568.
4. Field PA. The impact of nursing theory on the clinical decision making process. *J Adv Nurs.* 1987;12:563-571.
5. Garrett B, Callear D. The value of intelligent multimedia simulation for teaching clinical decision-making skills. *Nurse Educ Today.* 2001;21:382-390.
6. Hercelinskyj G, McEwan B. The Charles Darwin University vHospital: creating an authentic virtual learning environment for undergraduate nursing students. In: Keppell N, ed. *Physical and Virtual Learning Spaces in Higher Education.* Hershey: IGI Global; 2011.
7. Hughes M, Ventura S, Dando M. On-line interprofessional learning: introducing constructivism through enquiry-based learning and peer review. *J Interprof Care.* 2004;18(3):263-268.
8. Langford S. The Royal Flying Doctor Service of Australia: its foundation and early development. *Med J Aust.* 1994;161(1):91-94.
9. O'Connell B, Macdonald K, Kelley C. Nursing handover: it's time for a change. *Contemp Nurse.* 2008;30:2-11.
10. Reilley DE, Oermann MH. *Clinical Teaching in Nursing Education.* New York: NLN Publications; 1992.
11. Rees RS, Bashshur N. The effects of TeleWound management on use of service and financial outcomes. *Telemed J E Health.* 2007;13(6):663-674.

Telenursing: Current Scenario and Challenges for Brazilian Nursing

3

Isabel Amélia Costa Mendes, Simone De Godoy, Carlos Alberto Seixas,
Maria Suely Nogueira, Maria Auxiliadora Trevizan, Leila Maria Marchi Alves,
Elaine Maria Leite Rangel, and Alessandra Mazzo

Abbreviations

BIREME	Latin American and Caribbean Centre for Health Science Information
CNPq	Brazilian National Council for Scientific and Technological Development
EERP	Ribeirão Preto College of Nursing
GEPECOPEn	Study and Research Group on Communication in the Nursing Process
HCFMRP-USP	University hospital of the University of São Paulo at Ribeirão Preto Medical School
ICN	International Council of Nurses
ICT	Information and Communication Technologies
NTP	National Telehealth Program
SAS	Secretary for Healthcare
SEED	Secretary of Distance Education
SESu	Secretary of Higher Education
SGTES	Secretary for the Management of Health Work and Education
SUS	Unified Health System
USP	University of São Paulo
WHO	World Health Organisation

3.1
Background Information

In Brazil, the development of telenursing started in the year 2000, with the pioneer work of the Study and Research Group on Communication in the Nursing Process, GEPECOPEn. This research group at the University of São Paulo (USP) at Ribeirão Preto College of Nursing, EERP, a WHO Collaborating Centre for Nursing Research Development, has

I.A.C. Mendes (✉)
University of São Paulo, Ribeirão Preto College of Nursing, Avenida Bandeirantes, 3900
14040-902, Ribeirão Preto, Brazil/São Paulo, Brazil
e-mail: iamendes@usp.br

S. Kumar and H. Snooks (eds.), *Telenursing*, Health Informatics,
DOI: 10.1007/978-0-85729-529-3_3, © Springer-Verlag London Limited 2011

worked on projects that can optimize physical, technological, and human resources in health promotion actions at the interface between research, teaching, and permanent – in-class and distance – education by using communication technologies.

Historically, Brazilian nursing is characterized by a lack of technological resources for multi-disciplinary actions, without the need for displacement of all partners involved in research, teaching-research, or permanent education project.[9] In addition, the Brazilian health-care context is going through intense changes in its structure, in the conception of the health system and in the preparation of human resources. This scenario has benefited the development of telehealth in Brazil and allowed nursing to incorporate education technologies in human resource training and permanent education.

In a time marked by scarce resources, telenursing can and should use existing structures within colleges to a maximum in the training and development of nursing human resources among institutions in the same country and among countries, bringing teachers and students closer while enriching and strengthening the learning experience.

As a result of a review and analysis of this innovation, ICN published international competencies for telenursing, recommending the use of these competencies in the context of professional development, organizations, ethical and legal practice, and patient safety.[6]

3.2
Telehealth and Telenursing in Brazil

The Ministry of Health is responsible for the Health Education Policy, which includes the use of modern information and communication technologies to qualify health care. In 2007, it established the National Telehealth Program, NTP, aimed at developing health-care support and, mainly, permanent education within the Family Health Program, a strategy to consolidate the Unified Health System, SUS, which is the Brazilian public health system. The goals of NTP actions are education for work and, in the perspective of changes in work practices, the quality of basic health-care services within the SUS.[1]

The development of the NTP is part of a wide range of governmental actions coordinated by the Ministry of Health, through its Secretary for the Management of Health Work and Education (SGTES) and its Secretary for Healthcare (SAS), also involving the Ministry of Education (Secretaries of Higher Education (SESu) and Distance Education (SEED)), Civil Cabinet, the Pan American Health Organization, the Ministries of Science and Technology, Defence and Communications, besides different public universities and organizations like the Latin American and Caribbean Centre for Health Science Information, BIREME, the Federal Council of Medicine, and the Brazilian Society of Family and Community Medicine. The program aims to integrate family health teams across Brazil with academic reference centers, so as to improve primary health care by decreasing health costs through professional qualification, reducing unnecessary patient displacement, and increasing disease prevention activities.[1]

In Brazil, telenursing has emerged as a branch of telehealth and was recently included in the NTP by the creation of telenursing centers in some Brazilian states. Despite the wide range of possibilities the use of telematics resources can offer for professional health practices, literature shows that, in Brazil, telenursing development has been stronger in tele-education, with permanent education programs in nursing and health[4,5,7,8,10,14] and the production of learning objects.[3]

In addition to this scenario, health (nursing, medicine, dentistry, etc.) education is going through a reorientation process, working to prepare professionals who are skilled to respond to the Brazilian population's actual health needs and to put the SUS in practice.

Against this background, we will briefly describe the telenursing work of GEPECOPEn.

3.3
GEPECOPEn: A Pioneer in Brazilian Telenursing

A fundamental lever for GEPECOPEn to start its telenursing activities was the funding it received from the Brazilian National Council for Scientific and Technological Development, CNPq, in 2000, for a project called "Virtual Nursing, Research & Distance Education, Human Resource Training & Development."

The creation of this project was a result of the research group coordinator's concern with the lack of privacy patients are exposed to at different health institutions in practical learning situations. The coordinator started to look for technological resources to make the clinical learning environment more humane. The project consisted in the development of a video, audio, and data communication system for the simultaneous transmission and reception of multimedia information between two institutions – a nursing college and a university hospital – located on the same campus, so as to support research and innovations in nursing teaching.

The project was elaborated through PC-based videoconferencing technologies, using Polycom View Station videoconferencing equipment. While dealing with infrastructural and network aspects of such a novel undertaking, the group presented the project to the board of the Hospital das Clínicas, the university hospital of the USP at Ribeirão Preto Medical School, HCFMRP-USP. The research proposal was analyzed in detail by legal and ethical instances because images of patients, professionals, researchers, and faculty members would be transmitted.

GEPECOPEn assumed the ethical commitment that all projects involving the use of videoconferencing equipment should include the use of free and informed consent terms with the following aspects:

1. Participants should be aware that their image will only be transmitted in the academic–scientific context, including their face when transmission is online and filming cannot be avoided.
2. Participants should be aware that the authorization to use their image and the transfer of copyright do not oblige EERP, HCFMRP, or the USP in any way.

Moreover, it was established that, whenever any person's face did not have to be filmed, this should be avoided and, if this was impossible, images that could identify that person would be edited to use the material "offline."

After installation of the equipment and training for system operation and maintenance, a workshop was held for the scientific and technical community at USP, demonstrating all system characteristics and potential for expansion.

During this workshop, a medication administration procedure carried out at the hospital was simultaneously transmitted, through videoconferencing, to workshop participants at EERP. An undergraduate student simulated being a hospitalized patient who received the medication. Demonstrating nursing procedures is a widely used teaching strategy for traditional teaching in nursing laboratories or clinical contexts but can only be used with small groups of students.[9]

At the end of the demonstration, a workshop participant asked the student about the experience as a "patient." According to the student: *the experience was valid, because you do not expect everyone to be watching, although you know about the audience on the other side. The environment was calmer, without snooping looks.* About the academic experience, the student considered that *sometimes, as there are many people standing around the bed during the procedure, you cannot see it properly. Through videoconferencing, it is much easier for students on the other side to watch the procedure.*

As a result of this experience, the use of videoconferencing technology was incorporated into undergraduate nursing teaching as a support resource for in-class teaching in clinical situations between laboratories at the same institution, between the hospital and the college and between the college and other health institutions in São Paulo state.

3.4
Education and Training Opportunities

Besides applications in undergraduate teaching, videoconferencing technology has also been used for in-service training of nursing workers about intramuscular medication administration in the ventrogluteal region.[4]

A study of training offered to 30 nursing auxiliaries involved, besides classes through videoconferencing, on-site training and assessment of motor skills in simulated situations, and an opinion survey about the technology used.

In response to a questionnaire on the use of videoconferencing as a resource of in-service health education, students' evaluations were highly positive. When asked about their motivation to watch a distance education class through videoconferencing, the students highlighted the facility to conciliate work with in-service education and the opportunity to participate in an innovative strategy. All but one student felt motivated to discuss the contents learned during and/or at the end of the class.

Although research in this area is incipient, the above study showed that videoconferencing is a good learning facilitator. The possibility to conciliate work with training was important, as it avoided shift changes or work during free time. This may have influenced motivation for learning and satisfaction about technology use.

The fact that most participants indicated that they remained concentrated during the entire class is noticeable, as students tend to lose their concentration on the videoconferencing equipment after less than 15 min of class, so that distance education teachers have to seek other forms of interaction.[13] This highlights the importance of exploring all videoconferencing resources and incorporating them into training programs, granting professionals who are located distant from training sites access to new knowledge.

The above research provides evidences supporting the capacity of videoconferencing to optimize actions to promote permanent education at a distance, mainly in large countries like Brazil. At the time of study, no reports of similar courses or training were found in Brazilian literature, which makes this research another landmark for Brazilian telenursing.

Despite the success of the videoconferencing projects, GEPECOPEn felt the need to incorporate a virtual learning environment into its projects, which permits a broader space for in-service education and offers professionals access to learning objects at any time, independently of their work routine.

The project called "Researchers joining for Permanent Education in Health: Developing competencies, producing evidence, promoting change and innovation in health services" is funded by the Ministry of Health (SGTES) and partially guaranteed data network and equipment infrastructure conditions in a health district of Ribeirão Preto, a city of approximately 550,000 inhabitants in São Paulo state, under the responsibility of USP.

This project joined four health units with the university to develop health education actions. Each unit received a work station with a "thin client" (terminal for access to the virtual learning environment), keyboard, monitor, mouse, and a multipoint videoconferencing station.

Figures 3.1–3.4 show of one of the workstations to access the virtual learning environment and of a videoconferencing session between EERP-USP and one of the participating health units, distant 21 km from the university, where training was offered about hand washing.

In addition to the telenursing projects described above, GEPECOPEn innovated again by creating a course subject on telenursing in 2006. The subject is offered every other year to Bachelor and Teaching Diploma students at EERP. Its goal is to present technological advances in informatics and telecommunications, with a view to nursing students' adaptation to the reality of technology use in health care and education. Course contents include concepts of telemedicine and telenursing, with examples of Brazilian and international initiatives, presentation of information technologies involved in these initiatives, and discussion of infrastructure and operating aspects.

An analysis of students' expectations in taking the telenursing subject revealed four main areas, in order of relevance: using information and communication technologies, technological training for the labor world, getting to know telenursing and its resources, and improving nursing communication and care. Below are some examples of student expectations.

Fig. 3.1 Nursing worker accessing the virtual learning environment during her work shift

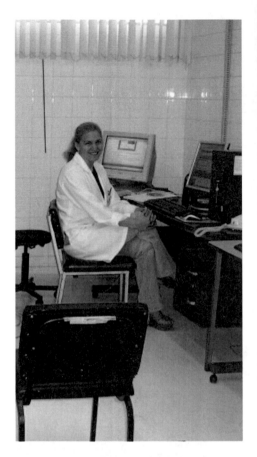

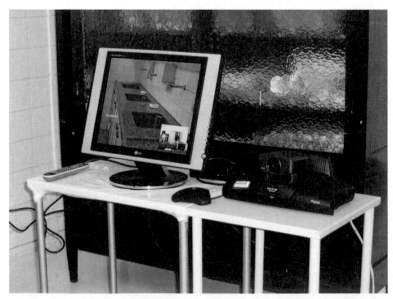

Fig. 3.2 Videoconferencing equipment already connected with clinical practice laboratory at EERP-USP

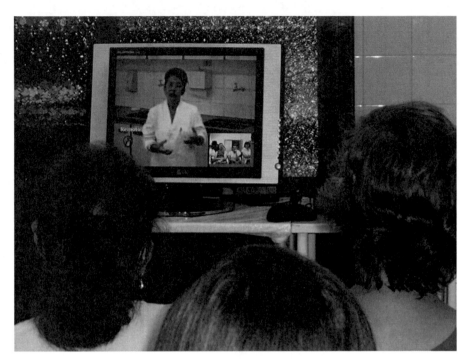

Fig. 3.3 Professor at EERP interacting with workers at the health unit

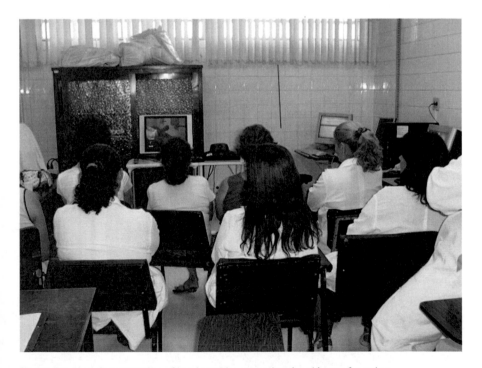

Fig. 3.4 Practical demonstration of hand washing procedure by videoconferencing

3.4.1
Using Information and Communication Technologies

- Adapting to needs related to new communication technologies
- Expanding knowledge on distance education
- Getting to know and using technologies

This category of expectations shows the changing roles these students perform, revealing a profile marked by greater initiative and competence for more autonomous and independent learning.

It is inferred that stimulating and exploring these characteristics in these students' training process can help incorporate the use of these communication technologies in professional nursing practice and strengthen nursing knowledge in line with current tendencies.[8] This is fundamental for professionals to act in a society marked by accelerated knowledge production.

3.4.2
Technological Training for the Labor World

- Learn the main methods of computer and technological communication to improve daily professional work.
- Learn and understand concepts in the course and apply them in daily professional routine.
- Develop/improve computer and communication knowledge in nursing.

This category shows students' perception about computer and technological recourse usage skills as a valuable component for professional practice. Their expectations evidence that they want to be professionals adapted to the needs of the job market in health.

3.4.3
Getting to Know Telenursing and Its Resources

More than any other sector linked to scientific and technological knowledge, computer and communication technologies are areas that have been undergoing rapid changes in this century. This premise, that is to offer students the possibility of contact with the application of telenursing resources as early as the beginning of the course, will grant them a differential in terms of knowledge about potential applications of these technologies, not only in their future activity areas but also during their training process.

It is important for nurses to understand how information technology can change their daily work and how they can use its benefits to create new processes of change.[2]

The expectations transcribed below evidence this context:

- Understand what telenursing is, where it is used, how professionals use it.
- Know the scope of telenursing around the world.
- Know what technologies are available to health professionals.

This category shows that the theme arouses the students' curiosity and stimulates them to seek knowledge and discover novelties through a course subject.

3.4.4
Improving Nursing Communication and Care

- Know how telenursing can interfere in patient treatment and care.
- Use telenursing to ease nurses' communication with the multi-professional team.
- How these resources can favor communication between professionals and patient education.

Expectations in this category show that students acknowledge the importance of communication for nursing care, feel the need to expand the possibilities and efficiency of this communication, and search for technologies to improve the nursing communication system. They also demonstrate that they perceive technological resources as ways to "interfere," "ease," and "favor" their professional practice, ranging from patient care to their multi-professional work. The need for technology-mediated communication skills to decrease related problems is evident.

The survey presented above is limited, as some points were not explored further or were lost when dividing the expectations into categories. Nevertheless, it indicates converge between the course contents and the students' expectations. Results value the role of education institutions to facilitate and offer students access to technological tools they will use in their job.

Educators need to take great care with student experiences during their training, as the desire to apply their learning in practice in the future depends on the preparation and education they are offered during their undergraduate program.[15]

In 2008, a new research project started, aimed at developing software to produce virtual models. These will be used to produce reusable learning objects in health. Infrastructure will be developed to elaborate animated demonstrations of nursing procedures and techniques, for use in health training and permanent education programs.

3.5
Discussion and Future Directions

Information and Communication Technologies (ICT) are present and influence all sectors of life. Today, it is hard to imagine any activity without them. Moreover, the job market in the twenty-first century demands permanent professional education to cope with complex and unforeseeable situations.

Nowadays, different organizations have used distance education to expand educational opportunities, offering students information access anytime and anywhere.[12] For nursing, distance education can enable professionals to prepare themselves and face the rapid changes of modern society, empowering them to manage their education throughout their lives.[11]

In Brazil, nursing has already moved beyond the stage of "discovering" the importance of using informatics and ICT for telenursing practice. The use of these technologies still remains mainly limited to administrative and educational activities.[4] Nevertheless, nursing is accompanying developments that point towards new professional activity areas.

In this context, the authors recommend that the use of these technologies be expanded to support teaching, care practice, and permanent education of health professionals. GEPECOPEn projects represent initiatives in this direction.

Currently available ICT reveal new forms of care delivery, taking into account professional needs and collaborating to change local, national, and international care practices by offering educational opportunities without the need for displacement from health services.

3.6
Summary

- In Brazil, the development of telenursing started in the year 2000, with the pioneer work of GEPECOPEn in the field of telenursing.
- In 2007, the Ministry of Health established the National Telehealth Program, NTP, aimed at developing health-care support, which also included telenursing.
- GEPECOPEn started telenursing activities with the project "Virtual Nursing, Research & Distance Education, Human Resource Training & Development," which was elaborated through PC-based videoconferencing technologies.
- GEPECOPEn incorporated a virtual learning environment into its projects. The project "Researchers joining for Permanent Education in Health: Developing competencies, producing evidence, promoting change, and innovation in health services" joined four health units with the university to develop health education actions.
- GEPECOPEn also created a course subject on telenursing in 2006, the course content including concepts of telemedicine and telenursing.

Glossary

Polycom view station – High-performance videoconferencing equipment from the manufacturer Polycom, used in the projects.

Thin client – Is a client computer in a "client–server" network. In the case of the research group's projects, it is a computer allocated at the health services with few applications installed, only those necessary to access the virtual learning environment installed on a server located at EERP-USP.

Ventrogluteal region – Region used for injectable medication administration through the intramuscular route.

References

1. Brasil. Biblioteca Virtual em Saúde. Telessaúde Brasil. Programa Nacional de Telessaúde em apoio à Atenção Básica. Disponível em: http://telessaude.bvs.br/tiki-index.php?page=Programa+ Nacional Acesso em: 15/01/2010. 2007.
2. Évora YDM. Nursing in the age of informatics. *Rev Eletr Enf.* 2007;9(1):14.
3. Franco E, Faculdade São Camilo. Escola de Enfermagem da USP utiliza a Telessaúde para a melhoria do ensino. Disponível em http://www.telessaude.org.br/noticias/noticia.aspx?ID= 1005953 [acesso 3/abril/2009]. 2008.
4. Godoy S, Mendes IAC, Hayashida M, et al. In-service nursing education delivered by video-conference. *J Telemed Telecare.* 2004;10(5):303-305.
5. Godoy S, Nogueira MS, Hayashida M, et al. Administração de injetáveis intramuscular na região ventroglútea: avaliação após treinamento por videoconferência. *Rev Rede Enferm Nordeste.* 2003;4(1):86-92.
6. ICN. *Standards and Competencies: International Standards for Telenursing Programmes.* Genebra: ICN; 2001.
7. Marin HF. New frontiers for nursing and health care informatics. *Int J Med Inform.* 2005;74:695-704.
8. Marin HF, Cunha ICKO. Perspectivas atuais em informática em enfermagem. *Rev Bras Enferm.* 2006;59(3):354-357.
9. Mendes IAC, Costa AL, Godoy S, et al. Grupo de pesquisa, difusão de conhecimento e EAD: um caso da enfermagem. In: Terra JCC, ed. *Gestão do Conhecimento e E-learning na prática.* 1st ed. Rio de Janeiro: Elsevier; 2003:285-293.
10. Peres HHC, Kurcgant P. O ser docente de enfermagem frente ao mundo da informática. *Rev Latinoam Enferm.* 2004;12(1):101-108.
11. Saback MAMC. A educação a distância como possibilidade para repensar as práticas educati-vas do enfermeiro frente às mudanças na sociedade contemporânea. *Sitientibus.* 2004;30(1): 21-30.
12. Schlemmer E. Metodologias para educação a distância no contexto da formação de comuni-dades virtuais de aprendizagem. In: Barbosa RM, ed. *Ambientes virtuais de aprendizagem.* Porto Alegre: Artmed; 2005:29-49.
13. Schneider MCK. *Distance Education: Challenges for Virtual In-Class Interaction Based on Technological Transfer in Videoconferencing Projects* [dissertation]. Florianópolis (SC): Graduate Program in Production Engineering/UFSC; 1999.
14. Seixas CA, Mendes IAC, Godoy S, et al. Implantação de sistema de videoconferência apli-cado à ambientes de pesquisa e de ensino de enfermagem. *Rev Bras Enferm.* 2004;57(5): 620-624.
15. Siler B, Kleiner C. Novice faculty: encountering expectations in academia. *J Nurs Educ.* 2001;40(9):397-403.

Telehealth Nursing in Canada: Opportunities for Nurses to Shape the Future

4

Antonia Arnaert and Fiona Macfarlane

Abbreviations

CDM	Chronic Disease Management
CNA	Canadian Nursing Association
EHR	Electronic Health Records
ICT	Information and Communication Technologies
IVR	Interactive Voice Response
NIFTE	National Initiative for Telehealth Guidelines
NP	Nurse Practitioner
RN	Registered Nurse
THN	Telehealth Nursing

4.1 Introduction

The publicly funded health-care system in Canada, known as "Medicare," has long been a source of national pride. The system, funded primarily by tax dollars, provides universal coverage and is based on the five principles of universality, portability, comprehensiveness, accessibility, and public administration.[36] Governed by the Canada Health Act, which includes the definition of the regulatory and funding schemes, the national health insurance program is composed of ten provincial and three territorial health insurance plans. Each province and territory is responsible for the management, organization, and delivery of health and health-care services to its residents[32] (see Fig. 4.1).

Canadians count on quality health care[35]; however, having access to quality care means accessing the right care, at the right time, by the right health-care providers, in the right setting. In recent years, the system has come under tremendous stress. The growing

A. Arnaert (✉)
School of Nursing, McGill University, 3506 University Street, Wilson Hall,
Montreal, QC H3A 2A7, Canada
e-mail: antonia.arnaert@mcgill.ca

S. Kumar and H. Snooks (eds.), *Telenursing*, Health Informatics,
DOI: 10.1007/978-0-85729-529-3_4, © Springer-Verlag London Limited 2011

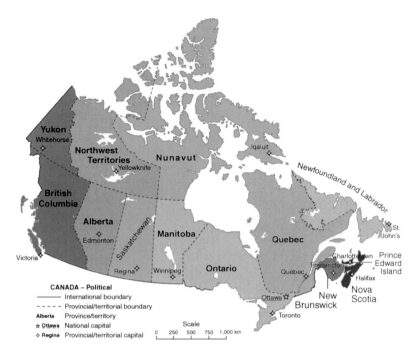

Fig. 4.1 Political Map of Canada: Province and territories

number of Canadians living with chronic diseases, an aging health-care workforce, changing patterns in health services delivery, the baby boom generation, and slow uptake of new technologies, such as electronic health records (EHR), are all affecting Canadians' access to health care.[6] Since publicly funded health care began in Canada, health-care services and the way they are delivered have changed from a reliance on hospital care to a focus on care in primary and community health centers, and homecare, as they are viewed as cost-effective alternatives to hospitals. Canadian health-care reforms also have placed greater emphasis on promoting health and wellness, preventing illness and managing chronic diseases, and increasing coordination and integration of comprehensive health-care services.

One of the most promising developments in health care today is the growing use of information and communication technologies (ICT) to provide information, assessment, and treatment to people with health concerns. This new field, known as "telehealth," has expanded greatly in Canada due to decentralization of health-care delivery and budgets.[22,35] No consensus exists on the definition of telehealth.[46] Industry Canada's Advisory Council on Health Infostructure has defined telehealth as "the use of ICT to deliver health and health-care services and information over small and large distances."[40] The term telehealth is often used alongside with "e-health," which is intended to be a more encompassing term. It covers an array of ICT applications, for example telehealth, health informatics, EHR, etc.[15] We will use the term telehealth throughout this chapter.

Telehealth practice spans all health disciplines. However, closely associated with telehealth is the term "telemedicine," which generally reflects the provision of physician-based health services. The literature defines "telehealth nursing" (THN) as "the delivery, management and coordination of care and services provided via telecommunication technology within the domain of nursing."[49] THN is a broad term encompassing all types of nursing interventions delivered across distances, which incorporate a vast array of telecommunication technologies, such as telephone, Internet, email, monitoring, and interactive video.

There is considerable evidence that THN can decrease the cost of patient care while improving the quality and access to care and patient satisfaction. In addition, used appropriately, telehealth has been shown to increase the productivity of nurses and their satisfaction.[49] Yet it is also known that many nurses and nursing managers have limited knowledge of current telehealth modes, programs, and outcomes. Hence, for the purpose of this chapter we have conducted 17 telephone interviews with telehealth nurses, coordinators, and experts in the field of THN across Canada and with resources from the provincial Colleges of Registered Nurses and/or College of Nurses to explore their views, perceptions, and vision of THN in Canada today and for the next few years. The phone interviews were guided by the following questions: How would you describe THN? What do you think are the competencies and qualifications needed for telehealth nurses? What do you think are the barriers and drivers for THN? What THN models do you use? What are the major policies' issues? How do you see the future of THN in Canada? Before presenting their insights it is important to understand how the nursing profession in Canada is regulated and the realities of today's nursing as it influences the practice of THN.

4.2
Canadian Nursing Regulatory Framework

In Canada the regulatory system for nursing reflects the country's federal, and provincial and territorial government structures.[16] Provinces and territories grant responsibility for regulation to professional colleges and/or nursing associations. Regulation means that certain nursing practice standards and rules are in place under specific legislation that governs the profession. It ensures that all Canadians who require nursing services will have a competent and ethical practitioner to provide it.[14] All provinces and territories have separate organizations, which regulate registered nurses (RNs) and other nursing categories, for example, registered practical nurses and registered psychiatric nurses. To ensure that RNs maintain their competencies to practice, regulatory bodies develop and govern continuing competency programs and set criteria for renewing registration.

Although the registration of nurses is done by the provincial and territorial regulatory bodies, the Canadian Nurses Association (CNA) is committed to advancing the discipline of nursing and the regulation of RN in the interest of the public. CNA works with the regulatory bodies to promote the development of regulatory approaches, which are coordinated, enhance accountability, and promote the mobility of RNs in Canada.[12] They provide the Code of Ethics for Registered Nurses to its member jurisdictions.[11] On a world stage, the CNA raises awareness of international factors that affect the regulation of nurses.

4.3
Today's Canadian Nursing Reality

According to the CNA, there were 252,948 RNs in Canada in 2006.[6] In terms of numbers, they comprise more than 25% of the health-care workforce.[5] Since 1998, the CNA has highlighted an impending shortage of RNs as it poses a serious threat to the Canadian health system.[7] Today, the CNA projects a gap between the supply of and demand for nurses at 78,000 RNs by 2011 and 113,000 RNs in 2016.[45] Increasing demands on the health system, an aging nursing workforce, cuts in the number of seats in nursing schools in the 1990s are all factors that will exacerbate this nursing shortage. Currently Canadian nurses are working 18 million hours of overtime every year – the equivalent of 10,000 full-time jobs. Health-care administrators, faced with the reality of different nursing compensation packages across the country, and young nurses disillusioned by poor working conditions have to deal with additional shortages as nurses migrate to better opportunities. In 2008, nurses in the province of Alberta had the highest wages in Canada with an average salary of $66,000, compared to the lowest average salary of $48,000 in the province of Newfoundland and Labrador.[41]

With the Canadian health system experiencing a physician shortage especially in rural areas, trends towards specialization in medicine with fewer physicians in primary care, and the changing role of the nurse from generalist to specialist, new areas of specialization have been developed and, in particular, the roles and duties of the RN have been expanded.[57] This expansion has created the role of nurse practitioner (NP), a title frequently used to identify advanced practice nurses. They perform tasks, such as inserting of arterial or central venous catheter, that have traditionally been considered the domain of physicians[23] and are now being viewed as a resource that can help to address gaps in the health-care system created by a physician shortage – a very economical solution given that these NPs are paid annual salaries of $80,000 versus $160,000 for physicians.[44]

It is clear that nursing and its regulation must evolve to adapt to the changing national and global environments and to meet the changing needs of all Canadians. Reducing the impacts of the nursing shortage can be achieved by reducing the health needs of the public and enhancing the availability of nursing services. In the following section, we will address how THN practice currently fits within the nursing profession in Canada and how it is positioning itself in the paradigm shift of traditional care models to emerging models of chronic disease management (CDM), patient self-management, and community-based patient and family-centered care.

4.4
THN in Canada

In this section, we discuss some of the initiatives and organizational bodies that have helped to shape the guidelines governing THN in Canada as well as some of the perceptions, thoughts, and ideas of telehealth leaders about THN. Their views are synthesized under the following headings: (1) THN guidelines – role of the CNA and provincial regulatory bodies, (2) today's THN delivery models, (3) competencies of telehealth nurses, (4) barriers and challenges to the expansion of THN, and (5) THN drivers and strategies for action.

4.4.1
THN Guidelines: Role of the CNA and Provincial Regulatory Bodies

The development of telehealth guidelines and specifically a national view of THN was driven by different groups responding to a need for leadership on issues related to tele-health and THN.

In November 2001, the CNA published its first position statement on "the role of the nurse in telepractice."[9] According to the CNA, nursing telepractice, which may also be referred to as "THN practice" and "telenursing," includes all client-centered forms of nurs-ing practice as well as the provision of information and education for health-care providers occurring through, or facilitated by, the use of telecommunications or electronic means. It is important to note that nurses engaged in tele-education are also considered to be engaged in THN.[8] Along with the position statement on THN, the CNA has a position statement around "nursing information and knowledge management" that reflects the role of nurses in man-aging information in health-care organizations. Together with leaders on health informatics, the CNA developed the "e-Nursing Strategy for Canada" in 2006, which explores the chal-lenges that face the nursing profession and elaborates on how information management and ICT can address those challenges.[13] e-Nursing refers to the incorporation of ICT into nurs-ing. The CNA Health Informatics Advisor described telehealth with EHR, decision support systems, and virtual learning environments as applications of nursing informatics.[30]

In 2000, the College of Registered Nurses of Nova Scotia published an initial set of telenursing practice guidelines to support nurses providing telephone support to patients living in rural and remote settings.[43] Ever since British Columbia,[19] Ontario,[18] Manitoba,[20] and Newfoundland and Labrador[3] have developed standards of practice for telephone and THN. Some provincial bodies still refer to the CNA THN guidelines for the standards applicable to their nursing membership. Another set of guidelines often referred to by the telehealth experts are the National Initiative for Telehealth Guidelines (NIFTE).[40] The NIFTE framework provides a structured set of statements to assist in the development of telehealth policy, guidelines, and standards. Since its publication in 2003, it has been used as a main source for the development of telehealth initiatives and has helped to anchor practice guidelines development by some provincial regulatory bodies.

One of the principles underlying safe, competent, and ethical THN is the principle of "locus of accountability." The CNA position statement on THN indicates that nurses engaged in telehealth are considered to be practicing in the province and/or territory where they live and are registered, regardless of where the patient is located. They must provide THN in agreement with the Code of Ethics, professional practice standards, relevant leg-islation, and practice guidelines of the province/territory in which they are registered and practicing. The College of Nurses of Ontario specifies in its guidelines that nurses regis-tered with the college may provide telepractice to patients in distance locations, including other provinces and countries.

4.4.2
Today's THN Delivery Models

Our communications with the telehealth experts helped us better understand the scope of THN practice across Canada, which is mainly concentrated with nurses providing telephone support and assisting during telemedicine encounters. "Home telehealth" is very new in Canada and unlike telephone nursing and telemedicine it is not yet recognized as a component in the provincial and territorial health systems and as such do not benefit from the vision, leadership, or health-care system funding that are available to the other telehealth domains. One expert who operates in Ontario specifically concentrated on the need for blending the telehealth services provided through telephone or other medium and telemedicine. Actually the expert emphasized the need for integration of telehealth in the current health system for the benefits of the patients, families, health-care providers, and the society in general. Currently many telehealth services in every province operate an isolated way.

4.4.2.1
Telephone Nursing

Telephone nursing is a subset of THN practice that involves giving telephone advice, usually after doing a tele-triage assessment, and often providing health referral information or education to callers.[28] Tele-triage is the process of assessing the priority of urgency of patient's symptoms by telephone.[51] Telephone nursing is not a new role for nurses. They have provided information, advice, and support over the phone for decades.

In Canada, most provinces and territories have 24/7 telephone nursing lines, which serve the entire population of their jurisdiction. These call centers, often called "Health Link" or "Info-Santé," are publicly funded and administered in Alberta, British Columbia, Manitoba, Saskatchewan, and Quebec. In contrast, the provinces of Ontario, New Brunswick, Nova Scotia, Newfoundland and Labrador, and the northwest territories have contracted out these services to private companies. Nurses providing telephone advice are using electronic protocols and/or guidelines to assess and manage patient symptoms. Some proponents saw these protocols as decision-making tools, others as decision-support tools. Telephone nursing is a rather inexpensive service for the government in regions where an entire population of a provincial jurisdiction can be reached with one service. With quite clear evidence that these services are safe and have high levels of caller satisfaction, governments are not waiting for evidence of effectiveness to move ahead with implementation. Evaluations to date in Canada showed minimal evidence of clinical impact and a cost per call ranging from $10 to $27.[51] Very few rigorous studies of these services have been completed. The studies that have been done show reductions in physician office visits, but there is no clear evidence of reductions in emergency room visits and this continues to be the subject of ongoing debate.[51]

Some interesting emerging care models for patients with a life-threatening and/or chronic illness are being developed and implemented in British Columbia and Manitoba via their public health lines. Since 2005, HealthLink BC[31] and the BC-Fraser Health Authority[26] have implemented an after-hour support system for end-of-life palliative patients and families. Patients and/or families can call the center after 9:00pm using a dedicated phone line, and the RN at HealthLink BC helps the caller using symptom management decision-making tools modified and adjusted to palliative and end-of-life care. The interface between the HealthLink and the Health Authority makes it possible to provide personalized palliative care to patients wherever they are and when needed.

In Manitoba, the Provincial Health Contact Centre has expanded their HealthLink scope to provide CDM. After patient enrolment, a comprehensive assessment is done that identifies how sick a patient is and how well patients are managing their chronic disease. The severity of the disease and patient level of self-management determine the level of support required, which subsequently determines the number of nurse contacts, education sessions, and data monitoring events that will be part of the patient's care plan. An interactive voice response (IVR) telemonitoring survey solution asks specific questions and captures vital sign data. Follow-up contacts with members of the health provider team are initiated as required. In Manitoba, this IVR system is also being used to support self-service education modules on a wide range of health issues and questions. In an effort to increase sustainability, the traditional health information/tele-triage model is evolving to offer proactive in-home care and in some cases may become the front line to the healthcare provider network.

4.4.2.2
Telemedicine Encounters

Over the past decades telehealth networks have been established in the majority of the provinces. These networks use videoconferencing technology (1) to provide clinical telemedicine services, (2) to provide continuing professional/medical education to health-care providers and the public, and (3) using telehealth equipment for administrative purposes.

Nurses play a key role in effective integration of telemedicine services and in the enhancement of satisfaction of both the patient and the physician with the outcome of the encounter. Some of the discussions we had with proponents in the field indicate that the role of the telehealth coordinator is not well defined and that the real scope of the role is often not well understood.

In most rural and remote settings, nurses and physicians determine whether a consultation with a specialist can be completed effectively using telehealth. In some communities an RN may not be available, so these communities rely upon someone other than a nurse to perform the telehealth coordinator role, which includes scheduling the appointment; educating the patient/family on the teleconsultation session, and overall equipment setup for the intervention. However, if a nurse is on hand at the distance site during the encounter, she/he will assist the physician specialist with the assessments, communicating key information and also serving as the patient's advocate. Prior to the scheduled telemedicine appointment time, the nurse will test the equipment, such as the examination camera, and have it ready at the time of appointment to save valuable consultant time. In addition, the nurse will review the concerns being addressed at the appointment and make sure to have all valuable information ready for the consultation, such as vital sign measurement, medications, and completed laboratory work. Patient and families are reminded what to expect from the encounter and how they can communicate with the specialist. During the consultation the nurse talks with the specialist and helps the patient and the specialist understand each other. After the teleconsultation, the nurse is advised of follow-up interventions as necessary and communicates these to the patient and other health-care providers.

4.4.2.3
Home Telehealth

Home telehealth defined as "the use of information, communications, measurement, and monitoring technologies to evaluate health status and to deliver health care from a distance to patients at home"[17] is not yet a part of the Canadian health system[24] regardless of its widespread recognition to potentially extend human resources, improve access to services, and minimize cost of care. The approach to home telehealth is very fragmented and, with the exception of Ontario, most are research-driven or isolated initiatives from local hospitals or treatment centers. Most are funded through special initiative government programs that are short term in nature and do not necessarily lead to program sustainability. Through the Ontario Telemedicine Network, Ontario has embarked upon the largest home telehealth program to date launching the "Ontario Telehomecare Program" which partnered with certain Ontario Family Health Teams. Currently about 600 patients are monitored remotely for CDM. Other home telehealth initiatives[2] vary in scope and size but involve a wide range of technologies from videoconferencing in the home to various models of telemonitoring and text-messaging devices. Health conditions being managed also vary greatly from CDM to short-term post-operative care, to oncology and palliative care symptom management. Telehealth nurses working in these programs are responsible for patient enrolment, ongoing symptom, and vital sign monitoring and management as well as the follow-up and referral to the broader patient health-care provider team.

4.4.3
Competencies of Telehealth Nurses

Nurses are committed to professional nursing practice that promotes quality, family-centered care, and efficient and effective delivery of integrated services provided by the members of a multi-disciplinary team.[27] Nursing has long prided itself on the values of compassion, provision of personalized care, and the ability to individualize care for different patients needs. In the last 50 years, however, nursing has been marked by tremendous change and nowadays they work in a variety of settings – in institutions, communities, and independent businesses – and fulfill diverse roles that require different skills and knowledge.

Currently a large number of nurses around the world are providing care via distance technologies, and in future telehealth will continue to expand the capacity of nurses to provide care to those with limited access to professional nurses.[37] Because the traditional laying of hands is no longer possible, telehealth nurses will need to develop complementary but different skills to use a broad range of technologies to support disease-management interventions for patients with chronic conditions and/or to assist physicians/physician specialists in telemedicine encounters with their patients. Clearly the question is "what complementary skills and knowledge must nurses have to incorporate new state-of-the-art technologies in their practice."[25] Before synthesizing the views of our proponents on this topic, it is clear that individual nurses are attracted to different kinds of nursing. McPhail[39] pointed out that the reason why nurses are attracted to a particular field is a result of their individual personality type. Results showed a correlation between nurse's level of educational preparation, numbers of years in practice, place of employment, and personality type.

4.4.3.1
Interpersonal Communication Skills

The effectiveness of an interactive two-way form of communication between a patient and a nurse is influenced by many factors such as the ease of operation and installation, picture/voice quality, and bandwidth. However, of equal importance is the nurse–patient interaction process. The way nurses present themselves on camera is extremely important and may indicate feelings of indifference, annoyance, or impatience. Nurses must try to establish "tele-presence" – the subjective sensation of "being there" in the remote location[34] – as they form relationships with patients and families. It is the skill of maintaining human quality in those relationships that will characterize the nursing profession in this rapidly advancing world of telehealth.[33] The American Nurses' Association[1] defined the required communication competencies of the telehealth nurses as follows: "Establish a therapeutic relationship which creates a sense of nursing presence that engages the client" and "assesses and adjusts communication techniques to maximize the nurse–client relationship."

4.4.3.2
Collaboration Skills

Telehealth may bridge gaps in the current health-care system between homecare, community, and tertiary care. However, this requires that nurses providing telehealth are knowledgeable about the different institutions, the providers to contact in case hands-on care is needed, but first and foremost they must be able to collaborate and feel comfortable working across disciplines and with different multi-disciplinary teams. Our experts often indicated the new role that local nurses in rural and remote centers or hospitals will have as they support physician specialists with their patients during a teleconsultation. The relationships for the local nurses will indeed change as they will need to work with different specialists, and in addition they will need to learn new medical specialties as patients post operation will be recovering from different types of surgical procedures and followed up at home.

4.4.3.3
Clinical Assessment Skills

Telehealth nurses must clearly have strong clinical assessment skills. They must be generalists with good basic skills and, as pointed out by our expert in Nova Scotia, telehealth nurses must be able to smell an emergency. Some employers, as indicated in the literature, require at least 3–5 years of experience in a variety of acute and/or community care settings before doing telehealth.[38] Nurses practicing THN must also be able to recognize if telehealth is appropriate or not to meet patients' needs and be able to support patients and families after the camera goes off.

4.4.3.4
Technology-Related Skills

It was clear to all proponents that telehealth nurses must have a positive and open attitude to the use of technology in general nursing practice. They must be knowledgeable about the technology they use in their practice and be able to troubleshoot certain technological issues. Everyone agreed that when a nurse is techno-savvy and has confidence using the technology, she/he will be able to teach and support the patients at home in using their monitoring and/or interactive video device or the health-care provider at the remote site during a telemedicine encounter. Information is key to effective decision making and integral to quality nursing practice.[10] Advances in ICT have accelerated efforts to implement information systems, and there is a need for all telehealth nurses to integrate nursing informatics competencies in their practice. Telehealth nurses must have strong computer and Internet skills as many of the remote monitoring applications are web based.

In summary, nurses are a key resource for health. They reach out to people with a continuum of care that is uninterrupted by time, distance, and setting whether in hospitals, in clinics, in community settings, in patient's homes, or through the use of telehealth. The skills and competencies needed as indicated above are subtle in nature. They are crucial to conducting successful telehealth visits – visits that will increasingly become a way of delivering nursing and other health services.

4.4.4
Barriers and Challenges to the Expansion of THN

While telehealth continues to evolve in every Canadian province, there are some real barriers that prevent the widespread implementation of THN. We summarized the barriers as follows.

4.4.4.1
Health-Care System Structures

The health-care delivery network in Canada is made up of many stakeholders and they vary from one province to another, all with their agendas and priorities. The telehealth framework adds a whole new set of telecommunications and technology partners to the health-care delivery system. This multitude of partners can lead to fragmented approaches that result in short-term models that cannot be sustained and changing and conflicting definitions of the THN role. Some experts voiced a concern that the role of the telehealth nurse could be defined by non-nursing members of the network. Gaining consensus around a telehealth vision and the required telehealth models will lead to a better understanding of the scope and the dimensions of THN. We also notice that despite the shift to more community and homecare, and the many initiatives taken by the federal and provincial governments to provide more continuity of care, interventions delivered to patients at home are still fragmented. Silos still exist from the acute care facility to the homecare support team, making integration across the multi-disciplinary health-care partners very limited.

4.4.4.2
Communication Infrastructure and Technology User-Friendliness

Access to broadband networks is still a major issue in most of the rural and remote communities in Canada. It seems, according to our experts, to still be an issue for the provision of telemedicine services in some remote regions and is a bigger problem for the delivery of home telehealth in those areas. Some patients have only dial-up connectivity at home and no broadband, which means that no interactive video sessions can be provided. Another point is the safety and user-friendliness of the many types of telemonitoring devices currently available on the market and their reliability in terms of accuracy and quality of data transferred by patients. Despite the ability of telemonitoring to provide timely data for nurses on the patient status, a complete understanding of how the data are collected and stored on host servers is minimal.

4.4.4.3
Data Security and Privacy

Linked with data reliability regarding submission and storage is the protection of patient privacy and personal health information. Not only must personal records be protected, but they must also be seen and believed by the general public to be totally safe from abuse or misuse. Because the electronic transmission of personal health information is the very underpinning of telehealth, it must be safeguarded through effective and enforceable privacy legislation and meticulous monitoring.[48]

4.4.4.4
Cost

The main concern today for the implementation and integration of home telehealth in the current health system is who will pay. Is home telehealth a cost-effective way of providing health care?[56] So far studies have focused on the patient outcomes, yet very few have examined telehealth from an economic cost perspective.[52] Many of the papers published to date on costs are anecdotal[33] or based upon only one homecare agency experience.[50] In addition, reported studies often used small sample sizes and the lack of robust economic analyses precludes generalization of financial results.[50] The most important factor for the use of home telehealth as indicated by our experts is a solid demonstration of its cost effectiveness, which is still unproven.[29]

4.4.4.5
Jurisdictional Issues

The nurse-centered locus of accountability adopted by the CNA and other nursing jurisdictions in Canada states that nurses practicing telehealth must be registered in the province where they work, regardless of the location of the patient. Despite this rule it appears to be an unresolved issue in provinces like Manitoba where the professional code for physicians is in direct conflict with the THN position statement. The questions are what are the implications for professional responsibility and liability? Who sets and enforces practice standards? And finally, who pays for the service?

4.4.4.6
Role Confusion and Credibility

While gaining more and more exposure, THN is still a largely unknown term for many within the health-care provider network, to say nothing of the general public. When asked about skill sets required to perform the THN role, all of our proponents were adamant that only nurses with a solid background in nursing could perform this role with one specifically saying that this is not a role for a new nurse. Lack of awareness and inconsistency of role definition for telehealth coordinators all contribute to create confusion and undermine the THN role and its credibility. The general public but also colleagues and other health-care providers need to understand the roles, responsibilities, and practice of THN.

4.4.4.7
Nursing Education in Telehealth

The lack of telehealth education is seen as a major barrier to nurses being able to acquire the necessary knowledge and skills to deliver telehealth. In 2002, Centennial College, Ontario,[53] was the first in Canada to build a modular online learning course for telepractice and telehomecare. No certification program exists in Canada, and no Center for Telehealth Nursing exists that is totally dedicated to THN development.

4.4.4.8
Shortage of Nurses

One of the greatest challenges the nursing profession faces, as mentioned earlier in this chapter, is the current and projected nursing shortages. There are not only shortages of nurses for specialty clinical areas and particular regions in Canada as in the past, but there are projected shortages that will affect all areas of our health-care delivery system,[54] including the provision of telehealth care that may be a solution for the shortages. As the human resource pool is not renewing itself at a sufficient rate because of practicing nurses retiring and an increasing number of nurses leaving the country,[47] there is no pool available from which to draw nurses for the practice of telehealth.

4.4.5
THN Drivers and Strategies for Action

The decentralization and fragmentation of health-care delivery, health budgets, and the population distribution have encouraged the development of telehealth across the country. Canada occupies the second largest landmass in the world and the population is concentrated close to the Canada–USA borders. Thousands of kilometers to the north of the country are relatively empty, embracing 41% of the land mass but only 0.3% of our population. Another driver to expand telehealth is the new generation of nurses and nurse students, who are entering the workforce or coming to school with iPods, cell phones, computer notebooks, and PDAs. The educational and health-care delivery system will need to make changes as they welcome young people long immersed in technology.

In the following section strategies for action and a vision of how NTH can move forward in Canada into the next decade will be defined.

4.4.5.1
Leadership and Vision Development

A vision of how nursing can move forward in the domain of telehealth can only be developed through a concerted effort by the members of the nursing profession across the country and the work done by special nursing interest groups from organizations, such as The Quebec Telehealth Network (Le réseau québécois de télésanté) and the Canadian Society of Telehealth. They are tackling many of the complicated issues relating to THN practice.

THN will be a critical component in the health-care delivery systems of the very near future. It is clear that to make THN a coast-to-coast reality for all Canadians, we need to have a national vision and unify our efforts, so that we can learn from each other and leverage the benefits.[48] Nurses may not sit back and wait for others to decide what the future should hold and how it can be affected. We need to invite ourselves into decision-making roles regarding THN. If we do not develop a future reality of our own then, as Porter-O'Grady[42] noted, anyone's future will do. Allowing others to plan nursing's future will serve neither the profession nor the Canadian society. We must take the initiative to demonstrate the value of THN and clearly articulate to the public the nature of THN and the differences it can make to the health and health care of all Canadians. It is clear that leaders in the area of THN must develop a collective conceptualization of its goals and develop a united front to accomplish them.[21]

4.4.5.2
Standards and Policies for THN Practice

It is the role of individual telehealth nurses, managers, and nursing associations to ensure that THN is provided in safe and healthy workforces. In addition, it is the responsibility of telehealth nurses to provide competent and quality care.[4] As this field further develops and becomes more central to health-care delivery, the treatment of ethical issues must be considered in relation to the society as a whole.[22] There is a need for policies that outline the mechanisms to protect patient information and accreditation standards defining who can provide THN and under which circumstances. Through the development of a professional THN framework in Canada, nurses practicing THN will feel proud of their profession and others will recognize and value the tremendous contribution that they make to the health-care delivery system.

4.4.5.3
THN Education and Learning Opportunities

THN should become an integral part of the nursing curriculum so that basic nursing education moves beyond thinking about technology-enhanced practice as an interesting aspect of future practice. The curriculum should include advanced assessment, communication and counseling skills, health informatics, ethics, and legal issues. Technology is a growing part of daily nursing practice and can only be expected to increase its scope of application in the future. In addition, ongoing professional development opportunities in THN and mentoring nurses now practicing in this field are extremely important.[40] Telehealth can provide opportunities for mid-career nurses and those with physical disabilities. However, it is imperative that we do not become dazzled by the potential of technology and as a result sacrifice the human touch.[48]

4.4.5.4
System Approach Within THN Practice

It is critical that Canadians become informed participants in the THN debate. Federal, provincial, and territorial governments can help facilitate the process of developing a shared, national vision. They can promote dialogue, educate consumers, and collaborate with the health care and professional organizations, institutions, and other stakeholders to develop the legal framework, standards, and policies, and the infrastructure needed to make THN a reality in Canada. Building networks and relationships with other care providers, government leaders, and policymakers will enable telehealth nurses to accomplish far more than we can by acting alone.

4.5
Conclusion

THN services, delivered over the phone or through other monitoring or interactive telecommunication devices to patients at home, are growing in the Canadian health-care system. Ultimately the marriage of these clinical nursing services with the services currently delivered in primary and community health-care centers, and homecare, would not only create new work life challenges and opportunities for nurses entering the nursing profession but also improve coordination and continuity of care, and thus patient quality of life. We invite nurses and nurse leaders to take the lead on the development of THN and its integration in the health-care system. While telehealth is certainly no panacea, we believe that technology, if used appropriately, may improve the health and health services enjoyed by all Canadians, no matter where they live.

4.6
Summary

- One of the most promising developments in health care in Canada is the growing use of "telehealth."
- THN encompasses all types of nursing interventions delivered across distances, which incorporate telecommunication technologies such as telephone, Internet, email, monitoring and interactive video.
- While telehealth continues to evolve in every Canadian province, there are some real barriers that prevent the widespread implementation of THN.
- A concerted effort by the members of the nursing profession can help promote the expansion and development of the THN role in the redesign of the Canadian health-care delivery system.
- Technology, if used appropriately, may improve the health and health services enjoyed by all Canadians, no matter where they live.

Acknowledgments   We would like to thank the telehealth nurses, coordinators, and experts in the field of telehealth in Canada for their insight and contribution. We also thank our contacts from the different nursing regulatory bodies in Canada for their views and thoughts about THN practice.

References

1. American Nurses' Association (ANA). *Competencies for Telehealth Technologies in Nursing*. Washington, DC: ANA; 1999.
2. Arnaert A, Wainwright M. Developing a home telecare service for elderly patients with COPD: steps and challenges. *Can J Nurs Inform*. 2008;3:49-83.
3. Association of Registered Nurses of Newfoundland and Labrador (ARNNL). *Telephone Nursing Care: Advice and Information [Guidelines]*. St. John's: ARNNL; 2002.
4. Baumann A, O'Brien-Pallas L, Armstrong-Stassen M, et al. *Commitment and Care: The Benefits of a Healthy Workplace for Nurses, Their Patients and the System. A Policy Synthesis*. Ottawa: Canadian Health Services Research Foundation; 2001.
5. Canadian Institute for Health Information (CIHI). *Workforce Trends of Registered Nurses in Canada, 2006*. Ottawa: CIHI; 2007.
6. Canadian Institute for Health Information (CIHI). *Health Care in Canada* [book on the Internet]. Ottawa: CIHI; 2008. Available at: http://secure.cihi.ca/cihiweb/products/HCIC_2008_e.pdf [cited July 20, 2010]

7. Canadian Nurses Association (CNA). *The Quiet Crisis in Health Care: A Submission to the House of Commons Standing Committee on Finance and the Minister of Finance.* Ottawa: CNA; 1998.
8. Canadian Nurses Association (CNA). National working group on nursing telepractice: draft report. Paper presented at: The Board Meeting of the Canadian Nurses Association; 2000; Ottawa.
9. Canadian Nurses Association (CNA). *The Role of the Nurse in Telepractice [Position Statement].* Ottawa: CNA; 2001.
10. Canadian Nurses Association (CNA). What is nursing informatics and why is it so important? *Nurs Now Issues Trends Can Nurs.* 2001;5:49-83.
11. Canadian Nurses Association (CNA). *Code of ethics for registered nurses.* Ottawa: CNA; 2002.
12. Canadian Nurses Association (CNA). *Accountability: Regulatory Framework [Position Statement].* Ottawa: CNA; 2005.
13. Canadian Nurses Association (CNA). *E-Nursing Strategy for Canada.* Ottawa: CNA; 2006.
14. Canadian Nurses Association (CNA). *Canadian Regulatory Framework for Registered Nurses [Position Statement].* Ottawa: CNA; 2007.
15. Canadian Nurses Association (CNA). *Telehealth: The Role of the Nurse [Position Statement].* Ottawa: CNA; 2007.
16. Canadian Nurses Association (CNA). Understanding self-regulation. *Nurs Now Issues Trends Can Nurs.* 2007;21:1-4.
17. Celler BG, Lovell NH, Chan DKY. The potential impact of home telecare on clinical practice. *Med J Aust.* 1999;171:518-521.
18. College of Nurses of Ontario (CNO). *Telepractice.* Toronto: CNO; 2005.
19. College of Registered Nurses in British Columbia (CRNBC). *Telehealth [Practice Standard for Registered Nurses and Nurse Practitioners].* Vancouver: CRNBC; 2005.
20. College of Registered Nurses of Manitoba (CRNM). *Telephone Nursing Care: Standards of Practice Application.* Winnipeg: CRNM; 2002.
21. Corcoran R. Nursing organizations face the future: will they survive? *Nurs Adm Q.* 2000;24: 52-53.
22. Cornford T, Klecun-Dabrowska E. Ethical perspectives in evaluation of telehealth. *Camb Q Healthc Ethics.* 2001;10:161-169.
23. Daly BJ. *The Acute Care Nurse Practitioner.* New York: Springer Publishing Company, Inc.; 1997.
24. Donahue M. Regulating telehealth in Ontario: next step in the transformation agenda. *Telehealth Law.* 2006;6:17-44.
25. Edirippulige S. Australian nurses' perceptions of e-health. *JTT.* 2005;11:266-268.
26. Fraser Health [homepage on the Internet]. Available at: http://www.fraserhealth.ca/ [cited July 20, 2010].
27. Girard F, Linton N, Besner J. Professional practice in nursing: a framework. *Nurs Leadersh.* 2005, 18(2), 1-8.
28. Goodwin S. Telephone nursing: an emerging practice area. *Nurs Leadersh.* 2007;20:37-45.
29. Håkansson S, Gavelin C. What do we really know about the cost-effectiveness of telemedicine? *JTT.* 2000;6:133-136.
30. Hannah KJ. Health informatics and nursing in Canada. *Healthc Inf Manag Commun.* 2005;19:45-51.
31. Healthlink BC [homepage on the Internet]. Available at: http://www.healthlinkbc.ca/ [cited July 20, 2010].
32. Houston K. Access denied: Canada's healthcare system turns patients into victims. *Policy Perspect.* 2003;10:6.
33. Hughes EM. Communication skills for telehealth interactions. *Home Healthc Nurse.* 2001;19:469-472.
34. Ijsselsteijn WA, de Ridder H, Freeman J, et al. Presence: concept, determinants and measurement. *Proc SPIE.* 2000;3959:520-529.

35. Jennett PA, Person VLH, Watson M, et al. Canadian experience in telehealth: equalizing access to quality care. *Telemed Health.* 2000;6:367-371.
36. Klatt I. Understanding the Canadian health care system. August 1–11, 2000. Available at: http://www.cfp-ca.org/learningcentre/The%20Canadian%20Health%20Care%20System.pdf [cited July 20, 2010].
37. Lamb GS, Shea K. Nursing education in telehealth. *JTT.* 2006;12:55-56.
38. McKession Canada Corporation [homepage on the Internet]. Available at: http://www.workopolis.com/EN/job/10834774 [5 June update 2009; cited July 20, 2010].
39. McPhail KJA. The nursing profession, personality types and leadership. *Leadersh Health Serv.* 2002;15:vii-x.
40. National Initiative for Telehealth. Framework of guidelines (NIFTE Guidelines). 2003. Available at: http://cst-sct.org/resources/FrameworkofGuidelines2003eng.pdf [cited June 12, 2010].
41. Ogilvie M. *Canada's Nursing Crisis Worse Than Ever.* Toronto: Toronto Star; 2008.
42. Porter-O'Grady T. A glimpse over the horizon: choosing our future. *Orthop Nurs.* 1998;17: S53-S61.
43. Registered Nurses Association of Nova Scotia (RNANS) [now the College of Registered Nurses of Nova Scotia]. *Guidelines for Telenursing Practice.* Halifax: RNANS; 2000.
44. Rogers D. Health care's new front line. *Ottawa Citizen,* October 2002.
45. Ryten E. *A Statistical Picture of the Past, Present and Future of Registered Nurses in Canada.* Ottawa: Canadian Nurses Association; 1997.
46. Schmeida M, McNeal R, Mossberger K. Policy determinants affect telehealth implementation. *Telemed Health.* 2007;13:100-107.
47. Sibbald J. Special news report. The future supply of registered nurses in Canada: a new study commissioned by the Canadian Nurse Association urges immediate action to avert a shortage. *Can Nurse.* 1998;94:22-23.
48. Siman AJ. Sharing the caring: telehealth offers fairer distribution of health expertise across Canada. *HCIM&C4th Quater.* 1999:12-14.
49. Sorrells-Jones J, Tschirch P, Liong MAS. Nursing and telehealth: opportunities for nurse leaders to shape the future. *Nurse Lead.* 2006;4:42-58.
50. Spetz J. The cost and cost-effectiveness of nursing services in health care. *Nurs Outlook.* 2005;53:305-309.
51. Stacey D, Hussein Z, Fisher A, et al. *Telephone Triage Services: Systematic Review and a Survey of Canadian Call Centre Programs.* Ottawa: Canadian Coordinating Office for Health Technology Assessment; 2003.
52. Stachura ME, Khansanshina EV. Telehomecare and remote monitoring: an outcomes overview. Report prepared for The Advanced Medical Technology Association. October 31, 2007. http://www.viterion.com/web_docs/Telehomecarereport%20Diabetes%20and%20CHR%20Meta%20Analyses.pdf
53. Telehealth centennial college, education opportunities: change management and knowledge transfer in E-Learning and E-Health [homepage on the Internet]. Available at: http://www.telehomecare.ca/education.html [cited July 20, 2009].
54. Thomlinson E, McIntyre M. The Canadian nursing profession: looking ahead. In: McIntyre M, Thomlinson E, eds. *Realities of Canadian Nursing: Professional, Practice, and Power Issues.* Philadelphia: Lippincott; 2003.
55. Whitten P, Kingsley C, Grigsby J. Results of a meta-analysis of cost–benefit research: is this a question worth asking? *JTT.* 2000;6:4-6.
56. Whitten P, Mair F, Collins B. Home telenursing in Kansas: patients' perceptions of uses and benefits. *JTT.* 1997;3:67-69.
57. Worster A, Sardo A, Thrasher C, et al. Understanding the role of practitioners in Canada. *CJRM.* 2005;10:89-94.

Telenursing in an Emerging Economy: An Overview

5

K. Ganapathy and Aditi Ravindra

Abbreviations

ASHA	Accredited Social Health Activist
CAPTOS	Child and Adolescent Psychological Telemedicine Outreach Service
CGFNS	Commission of Graduates of Foreign Nursing Schools
DIY	Do It Yourself
ECG	Electrocardiography
GDP	Gross Domestic Product
ISDN	Integrated Services Digital Network
NRHM	National Rural Health Mission, India
PDA	Personal Digital Assistant
VSAT	Very Small Aperture Terminal
WHO	World Health Organisation

5.1 Introduction

"Watson, come here I want you" said Alexander Graham Bell on 20 March 1876 when he inadvertently spilled battery acid on himself, while making the world's first telephone call. Little did Bell realize that this was also the world's first telemedical consultation.[12] Telemedicine has come a long way since then. Telemedicine, a method by which patients can be examined, investigated, monitored, and treated, with the patient and the health-care provider physically located in different places, is slowly becoming an integral part of the health-care delivery system. Using available hardware and telemedicine software, and establishing connectivity through ISDN lines, broadband, or VSATs (very small aperture terminals), tele-health is making distance meaningless and geography history!![13] Clinical information can be

K. Ganapathy (✉)
Apollo Telemedicine Networking Foundation, Apollo Hospitals, #21, Greams Road,
Chennai 600006, India
e-mail: drganapathy@apollohospitals.com

S. Kumar and H. Snooks (eds.), *Telenursing*, Health Informatics,
DOI: 10.1007/978-0-85729-529-3_5, © Springer-Verlag London Limited 2011

transmitted from peripheral medical devices. These include among others a stethoscope, a pulse rate monitor, a blood pressure monitor, and an ECG monitor. This clinical data could initially be evaluated electronically by a nurse at a remote place, making a "telenurse" the first point of contact in the health-care delivery system. Thus, unnecessary traveling of patients and their escorts to health-care centers could be eliminated.[15] It is in emerging economies, with limited resources, that telenursing can be predominantly beneficial. While telemedicine in some form exists in most countries in the global south, telenursing is still in its infancy. It was Victor Hugo who once remarked "There is nothing more powerful than an idea whose time has come." Perhaps the time is now ripe for telenursing.

The International Council of Nurses (2007) has defined telenursing as the use of tele-medicine technology, to deliver nursing care and conduct nursing practice.[34] Telemedicine in this case is defined as *tele* – "distance" and *mederi* – "healing," which encompasses the use of telephone, Internet, sensors, video, remote diagnostics, and/or other interactive technologies that allow interchange between patients and nurses or between nurses and other health-care providers. The Telenursing Working Group of the International Society for Telemedicine and e-Health has endorsed the necessity for the increased adoption of telehealth/telemedicine by nurses to ensure collaboration across disciplines (physicians, therapists, and other health-care team members) and with patients. Telenursing would also "export" nursing knowledge and expertise, using technology to those who need care, in accordance with the appropriate scope of nursing practice in the telenurses' country. Nurses are the single largest group of health-care providers internationally. Therefore, it is crucial that nurses are involved in the development, planning, implementation, and man-agement of telemedicine/telehealth and e-Health programs and policies at all levels.[34]

With telenursing becoming an expanding service in many western countries, the face of standard nursing practice is changing.[5,50] Telenursing offers help by assessing the health sta-tus of a caller.[41] It has often been hypothesized that it is easier to talk to a woman and hence telephone triage by women nurses is becoming well established. McDermott has reported on the reduction of costs and improved access to health care, for rural patients, through telenurs-ing.[48] Henderson has reported on distance emergency care in rural emergency departments using nurse practitioners.[25] With increasing availability of telenursing in an integrated health-care delivery system, legal issues are likely to emerge. Multi-state licensure is one such concern.[8] Studies in Québec to evaluate telenursing outcomes: satisfaction, self-care prac-tices, and cost savings have been reported by Hagan.[22] Satisfaction levels, specific knowl-edge and skills, telenurses' opinions on education in telehealth, their perceptions about the effectiveness of telenursing, and its future impact were reported in a survey of 719 nurses, from 36 countries, working with telehealth.[20] Telenursing in rural areas has also been shown to play an important role in Australia and other developed countries.[21,52]

5.1
Telemedicine in India

The Indian health-care industry is one of the biggest in the world, with every sixth indi-vidual on the planet being a consumer.[16] The doctor:population ratio is estimated to be 1:2,000. The Indian government spends only 0.9% of the GDP on health, of which probably 0.09% reaches the 700 million rural users.[2] Interestingly, the private sector dominates, by providing 80% of the health care. Despite establishing more medical colleges and recognizing several hospitals as post-graduate training centers, lack of doctors, specialists, and nursing and paramedical personnel continues to plague the system. Health care in India is indeed a paradox. While we are becoming the next global health tourism destination, with world-class centers of excellence, 700 million Indians have no direct access to secondary and tertiary medical expertise. Mahatma Gandhi once remarked "India lives in its villages." Seventy percent of the population, residing in rural areas, have limited access to medical care as 80% of the doctors live in the metros and the cities. On the other hand, the tele-density of India is growing exponentially. In January 2009 it was 34.5%.[30] In April 2011 it was 71%. Telecommunication infrastructure in rural India is today a reality (the rural tele-density in September 2008 was around 13%), which probably cannot be said about the availability of doctors and nurses.[37] Recognizing this, the public and the private sector have realized that telemedicine could possibly be the solution to bridge the gap in health services between the "haves" and the "have-nots."[13] Today, there are approximately 550 telemedicine units located in suburban and rural India,[18] seeking telemedicine consultation from specialists, in almost 70 tertiary care hospitals. It can be assumed that about half a million teleconsultations have probably taken place in India, the majority being in teleophthalmology.[4,49] The Apollo Telemedicine Networking Foundation, the largest and oldest multi-specialty telemedicine network in South Asia, has carried out about 68,000 teleconsultations in about 40 different specialties given to about 100 peripheral centers in India and overseas.

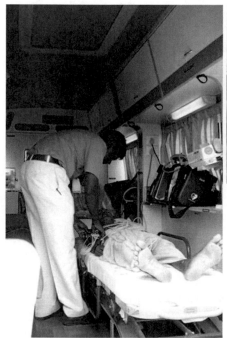
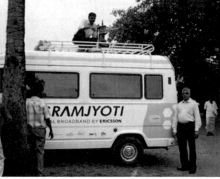

Fig. 5.1 Nurse transmitting clinical data from a village, through wireless-enabled van to a city-based consultant

Fig. 5.2 Advertisement of a
nurse station at an Apollo
pharmacy in India

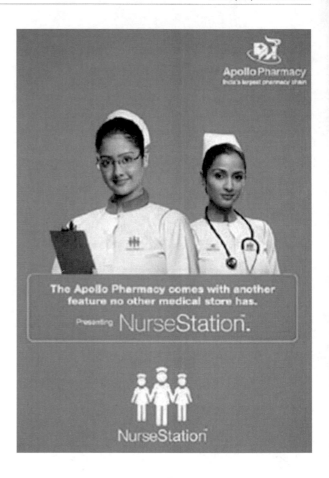

A unique method of reaching out to the masses in India is through the use of well-equipped "hospital-on-wheels." This has been most successful in the field of ophthalmology. Trained nursing assistants and nurses are deployed to towns to deliver ophthalmic care, supervised by consultant ophthalmologists from the metros and the bigger cities. VSATs, 3G, WiMax, and broadband are used for communication.[4,49] Nurse practitioners on hospital-on-wheels are the first level of contact with the patient (Fig. 5.1). This system is now increasingly being used in pediatrics, mental health, and diabetology. Telenursing in the field of mental health has also been described.[59]

The Apollo Hospitals Group, the largest health-care provider in Asia, has recently introduced an innovative program of making available nurses in selected Apollo pharmacies to facilitate health care (Fig. 5.2). It is proposed to link some of these pharmacies with the tertiary care center (Apollo Hospitals) through a telemedicine setup. A nurse stationed at the pharmacy would provide clinical information to a doctor and request for assistance. Trial runs have been carried out using a domiciliary telemedicine equipment to monitor blood pressure, ECG, and pulse rate of post-stroke patients. However, doctors were preferred at the hospital end instead of nurses. In March 2011 a 24/7 medical response center performing tele triage functions, predominantly saffed by nurses has commenced.

Table 5.1 Distribution of health service providers and nurses in WHO regions and the world

WHO region	All health service providers	Nurses	Nurses as % of health service providers
Africa	136,000	773,368	56.87
Americas	12,460,000	4,053,504	32.53
South-east Asia	4,730,000	1,338,029	28.29
Europe	11,540,000	6,526,461	56.56
Eastern Mediterranean	1,580,000	631,527	39.97
Western Pacific	7,810,000	2,903,286	37.17
World	39,470,000	16,226,175	41.11

Source: The World Health Report (2006)

5.2
Nursing Care in India

Out of the 2,300 institutions recognized by the Nursing Council of India to train nurses, 660 produce graduate nurses and 77 produce post-graduate nurses.[33] The Nursing Council of India needs to incorporate telenursing into the mainstream of nursing education and nursing care. This alone will give a fillip for the growth and development of telenursing. The nurse-per-bed ratio in India is 0.87 as against the world average of 1.2, based on WHO data. With attrition rates increasing, an acute scarcity of trained nurses is anticipated. Setting up of nursing colleges along with hospitals and integrating telemedicine technology into the nursing profession appear to be a plausible solution.[31] The first telenursing training center set up in Mysore, a city in southern India, is expected to increase efficiency and provide opportunities to medical and paramedical staff to enhance their knowledge.[31] Of the 30,000 nursing graduates produced every year, many take the CGFNS (Commission of Graduates of Foreign Nursing Schools) examination and obtain lucrative offers from abroad.[36] It is estimated that 2.4 million nurses will be required in India in 2012; however, a shortfall of 50% is expected. A 2006 World Health Report indicates that although the absolute numbers are very low, nurses constitute a sizeable portion of all health service providers. The ratio is particularly high in Africa as can be seen from Table 5.1.[38]

5.3
Telenursing in India: The Way Forward

Nurses constitute the backbone of health-care systems. It is important that they be trained to increase their reach and provide their expertise hundreds of miles beyond where they reside. When there exists an acute shortage of qualified nurses in urban India, it will be difficult to identify "telenurses." A telenurse needs to be a multi-faceted personality with excellent communication skills, be tech savvy, and have quick thinking ability with technical knowledge.

For telenursing to take off in India, awareness in the nursing fraternity is essential. Recently, a few nursing training centers have introduced telemedicine in their teaching program. For a successful outcome, evangelists to espouse and champion the cause are vital. It will take more time for traditional India to accept a telenurse – an individual competent to take independent clinical decisions. Telenursing involves sharing of clinical information with other professional colleagues, including national and international experts. Continuing nursing education programs will be easier. Clinical skills can be learned and practiced through patient simulation. Telenursing provides opportunities for experienced nurses to share their experience, without enduring the physical burden of "floor" nursing in hospitals.

A major incentive would be adequate compensation. In an Indian setting, it may not be easy to conceive and implement an innovative, self-sustaining, revenue-generating business model catering to all stakeholders. Development of a business model and integration of strategies with government plans are necessary. Issues such as driving force, target market, and expense sharing need to be examined in detail from both ideal and realistic points of view. Implementation strategies are crucial in ensuring that telenursing achieves the critical mass, essential for a successful take-off. Medical specialties where telenursing can function need to be identified. The necessity for verifying telenursing as a cost-effective health-care delivery system has been discussed.[63] Yun and Park, in a review of telenursing in Korea, classified other issues as systematic, economic, societal, and technical.[64] Development and regulatory challenges have to be considered.[23] Legal issues are equally important. The role of multistate registration to support nursing practice is described by Clark et al.[10] For a country like Australia, with a population of less than 250,000, having eight individual nurses acts probably suggests over regulation which may not be totally warranted.[10] However, for India, with the population reaching 1.2 billion, the need for stringent regulatory processes is eclipsed by lack of qualified health professionals. As individual state licensure for nurses is not mandatory at present, legal and regulatory issues will not be a deterrent.

5.4
Homecare

A distinctive telenursing application is homecare. Systems that allow home monitoring of blood pressure, blood glucose, respiratory peak flow, and weight measurement are now freely available in advanced countries. Immobile patients, those who live in remote or difficult-to-reach places, and those with chronic ailments (including chronic obstructive pulmonary disease,[61] diabetes,[43,44] congestive heart disease, or Parkinson's or Alzheimer's disease) could stay at home. They could be "visited," monitored, and assisted regularly by a nurse via videoconferencing. Wounds, ostomies, and immediate post-surgical situations can be electronically managed. Using telenursing, a nurse in the west electronically visits 12–16 patients instead of 5–7 per day. Call centers are operated by managed care organizations and staffed by registered nurses who act as case managers or perform patient triage, information, and counseling, as a means of regulating patient access and flow. This decreases visits to emergency rooms. Patient education and initial evaluation of results of medical tests and examinations could also be done. India, in the last few years, is witnessing well-trained qualified nurses providing care in a domiciliary setting. Traditionally in India, patients are more comfortable with formal nursing care than virtual visits. The scenario in many advanced countries is different. Through interactive video systems, patients can contact on-call nurses at any time. Instructions can be obtained on how to change a wound dressing, take an insulin injection, or manage an increasing shortness of breath. With increasing availability of "across-the-counter" home monitoring devices, blood pressure, pulse, and glucose monitors, the phrase DIY or "Do It Yourself" is becoming a slogan in health care. Nurses can provide virtual homecare, through accurate and timely information and support online. This ensures continuity of care. Allen et al. have demonstrated that telenursing visits could substitute for a substantial fraction of on-site home nursing visits. In the USA, employment in home health care is expected to increase 36% or more over the next 7 years. Forty-six percent of on-site nursing visits could be replaced by virtual visits.[1] Telenursing can reduce duration of hospital stays. In Denmark, hospital admissions and "bed days" reduced to 50% when nurses in a backpain clinic contacted patients telephonically. In another instance, in Iceland, a telephone-based nursing intervention supports mothers with difficult infants to reduce fatigue and distress. Innovative programs use telenursing to allow women with pregnancy-induced hypertension to remain at home.

The necessity of home telecare systems is growing owing to increase in chronic diseases, aged population (living alone), and medical expenses. It has been documented that a video visit is more cost effective in a geriatric population.[3,9] The progress of a post-operative wound or bed sore can be evaluated by a nurse through a digital photograph uploaded at home. Intelligent telephones can monitor vital functions from a distance. A nurse through a video surveillance unit can watch an elderly person,[60] instruct about taking pills, and even ensure that the refrigerator and pantry is adequately stocked. Borchers and Kee have opined that inexpensive domiciliary telenursing provides a method for early intervention.[7] Several publications have emphasized the facets of technology in home health care.[40,47,53] In Italy, specialized services for general practitioners, home telenursing for chronic patients, tele-diagnosis for palpitations, and call center services for hospitals are provided by many agencies, as in the Boario Home Care project.[55] Qualitative evaluation of an analogue videophone linked with a physiological monitoring device, in a home setting in Liverpool, was reported by Hibbert et al.[26] Clinical situations most amenable to telenursing included chronic airway obstruction and joint disorders. In a study in Belfast, two observers estimated that 14% of home nursing visits could be done via telemedicine, even with relatively low-quality compressed video.[62]

A call center triage is another important component in telenursing. On receiving a call, a trained nurse is expected to efficiently prioritize enquiries and get a physician's help when required. Studies are in progress, to understand how telenursing can be integrated into general practice.[58] Twenty-four-hour access to free telephone advice and symptom triage is available to residents in Australia and New Zealand. Nurse-led telephone help-lines across the UK have resulted in a necessity for the development of new nursing skills. Telephone nurses in Sweden assess care needs and provide advice, support, and information, recommending and coordinating health-care resources. New biomedical competence, an aging population, and constrained resources have made priority setting a primary concern. In an interesting study, Leclerc et al. cautioned that telephone health-line providers should be aware that many callers interpreted advice in a manner different from that intended.[45] Quality control interventions to reduce miscommunication and ensure better understanding will contribute to more effective service. Telephone-assisted problem solving by nurses, nurse-mediated SMS health alerts for vaccines, medication reminders, health checkups, health monitoring, diet, etc. are also part of the services offered in a call center.

Telenurses should be multi-faceted and competent in pharmacology, psychology, and communication. Telenurses also need training in handling overt or covert power messages based on male superiority. Training in technology to improve efficiency and recognition of the worth of *hands-on* nursing have been emphasized.[57] Telenurses at call centers often use decision aid software programs to offer triage recommendations and self-care advice to the general public.[27] At present sensitive decision-aid systems need to be developed exclusively for the global south.

With the exponential increase in telecommunications in emerging economies,[37] establishing telenursing call centers per se would not pose major difficulties. However, in the current cultural milieu, acceptability of this service could be an issue. Who would pay for such a service? Who would be legally responsible if errors are committed? Absence of uniform health standards further compounds the issue. The presence of 36 official languages, varying literacy levels, and diversity in social, economic, technological, and telecommunication development contributes to the complexities involved in introducing telenursing call centers in India. Telephone nursing has raised ethical questions. Conflicting values, norms, and interests are often encountered. In a multi-cultural society, ethical issues offer a challenge.[28,32]

5.5
Telenursing in Medical Specialties

Review of literature indicates that telenursing today is slowly being adapted to suit various medical specialties. With diabetes becoming endemic in most countries of the world, helping the diabetic patient to manage his/her condition is critical. In a study from Japan, significant improvements in levels of blood glucose and glycosylated hemoglobin (HbA(1c)) and in the patient's blood pressure were documented, when a telenursing system was used.[42] A child and adolescent psychological telemedicine outreach service (CAPTOS) started as early as 1997 has now shown to enhance the nursing care of young people with a complex mixture of psychological and physical health problems.[52]

Nursing care forms the *sine qua non* of hospice care, being a type and philosophy of care which focuses on the palliation of a terminally ill patient's symptoms. Telenursing is increasingly being used in hospice care. NurseLine, a telenursing system in hospice palliative care, achieved improved symptom management, decreased visits to emergency rooms, and provided enhanced support for families, caring for loved ones at home. Maximizing technology to create systems that improve access to care and are sustainable was one of the lessons learned.[51] In one study, it was documented that 64.5% of home hospice nursing visits could be substituted with a video phone. This reduction in personal visits significantly reduces the costs.[11]

Cardiology is an area where telenursing is deployed. Reports on effectiveness of structured, post-discharge, telephone intervention for patients recovering from bypass surgery and their partners revealed that timely reassurance and health promotion were possible.[24] One-lead electrocardiogram monitoring and nurse triage in chronic heart failure have been used in home telenursing.[54] Post-hospitalization telenursing care has shown to reduce readmission in cases of congestive heart failure.[39] Nurse-mediated PDA-supported decision support tools for cardiac tele-triage have recently commenced.

Oncology: In an outpatient management study of patients with cancer with new ostomies, patients believed that nurses had increased understanding of their problems. Patients were more comfortable communicating with nurses. Though telemedicine was preferred to waiting for face-to-face visits, the latter was still felt to be important.[6,46] Oncology nurses are best suited to transfer their expertise to patients and their health-care providers through telehealth technologies.[56]

5.6
Telenursing: A Different Approach for Emerging Economies

One of the key components of the Indian National Rural Health Mission is to provide a trained female community health activist in every one of the 600,000 villages in the country. Designated *ASHA* or *accredited social health activist*, she is selected from the village itself and is accountable to it. The ASHA is trained to work as an interface between the community and the public health system.[29] In pilot studies, the ASHA has been provided with a wireless PDA to establish contact with health-care personnel in the chain of command. This form of "telenursing" using innovative hi-tech communications for the field worker at the grass root level helps address the specific local challenges. Orissa, a less developed state in southeastern India, has effectively demonstrated that technology could be used in the collection of health data at the ground level. Under the Integrated Child Development Scheme, one *Anganwadi* worker is allotted to a population of 1,000. The duty of an Anganwadi worker is to ensure that regular health checkups, child development, adequate nutrition, immunization, health education, and non-formal pre-school education are made available. The data are entered in a PDA. With a click of the mouse, one can access the details of an Anganwadi worker and the children under her care, even if she is in the remotest corner of the state. However, not all hamlets in Orissa have an Anganwadi. This exercise in connectivity and the dissemination of information is becoming wireless. Mobile handheld units are being used in this project as data harvesting points for NRHM at the grassroots level.[19,35]

5.7
Issues and Challenges in Implementing Telenursing in an Emerging Economy

- Creating awareness and jobs and reducing brain drain.
- Acceptance of "telenursing" by nurses, society, patients, family physicians, specialists, administrators, and the government.
- Designing cost-effective appropriate need-based hardware, software, and connectivity for telenursing.
- Standardizing, certifying, authenticating, and registering telenursing units so that minimum safe standards are uniformly adopted.

- Introducing telenursing in the nursing curriculum and training the trainers.
- Recognition of telenursing by the National Nursing Council.
- Adequate reimbursement to make the scheme attractive and viable.
- Getting grants, subsidies, and waivers to introduce this in suburban and rural areas.

5.8
Conclusions

The challenge today is not confined to overcoming technological barriers, insurmountable though they may appear.[17] The take-off problem facing telenursing is legion. It is our dream and hope that within the next few years there will be telenursing units in many parts of India. Eventually a nurse should only be a mouse-click away!![14] Improbable Yes!! Impossible No!! For this to happen, a critical mass must be reached. What is required is not implementing better technology and getting funds but changing the mindset of the people involved. Awareness should permeate throughout society. Real growth will take place only when society realizes that distance is meaningless today and that telenursing can bridge the gap between the "*haves*" and the "*have-nots*," at least in so far as access to health care is concerned.

5.9
Summary

- Telenursing is the use of telemedicine technology to deliver nursing care and conduct nursing practice.
- A telenurse needs to be a multifaceted personality with excellent communication skills and quick thinking ability with technical knowledge.
- Telenursing today is slowly being adapted to suit various medical specialties. It is used in pediatrics, mental health, diabetology, cardiology, oncology, and hospice care.
- The tele-density of India is growing exponentially. Today, there are many telemedicine units located in suburban and rural India, seeking telemedicine consultation from specialists, and also about half a million teleconsultations have already taken place in India.
- One of the key components of the Indian National Rural Health Mission is to provide a trained female community health activist in villages, who is designated as ASHA and is trained to work as an interface between the community and the public health system.

References

1. Allen A, Doolittle GC, Boysen CD, et al. An analysis of the suitability of home health visits for telemedicine. *J Telemed Telecare*. 1995;5:90-96.
2. Annual Report 2007–2008. Ministry of Health & Family Welfare, Government of India. http://mohfw.nic.in/.

3. Arnaert A, Delesie L. Telenursing for the elderly. The case for care via video-telephony. *J Telemed Telecare.* 2001;7:311-316.
4. Bai VT, Murali V, Kim R, et al. Teleophthalmology-based rural eye care in India. *Telemed J E Health.* 2007;13:313-321.
5. Biedrzycki BA. Telenursing: nursing care without geographic boundaries? *ONS News.* 2005;20:9-10.
6. Bohnenkamp SK, McDonald P, Lopez AM, et al. Traditional versus telenursing outpatient management of patients with cancer with new ostomies. *Oncol Nurs Forum.* 2004;31:1005-1010.
7. Borchers L, Kee CC. An experience in telenursing. *Clin Nurse Spec.* 1999;13:115-118.
8. Brent NJ. Emerging legal issues for nurse managers. *Semin Nurse Manag.* 2000;8:220-225.
9. Chan WM, Woo J, Hui E, et al. The role of telenursing in the provision of geriatric outreach services to residential homes in Hong Kong. *J Telemed Telecare.* 2001;7:38-46.
10. Clark RA, Yallop J, Wickett D, et al. Nursing sans specialize: a three year case study of multistate registration to support nursing practice using information technology. *Aust J Adv Nurs.* 2006;24:39-45.
11. Doolittle GC, Whitten P, McCartney M, et al. An empirical chart analysis of the suitability of telemedicine for hospice visits. *Telemed J E Health.* 2005;11:90-97.
12. Ganapathy K. Telemedicine and neurosciences in developing countries. *Surg Neurol.* 2002;58:388-394.
13. Ganapathy K. Telemedicine in the Indian context. An overview. In: *Establishing Telemedicine in Developing Countries: From Inception to Implementation. Studies in Health Technology and Informatic,* vol. 104. Amsterdam: IOS Press; 2004:178-181.
14. Ganapathy K. Role of telemedicine in neurosciences. In: *Establishing Telemedicine in Developing Countries: From Inception to Implementation. Studies in Health Technology Informatics.* Amsterdam: IOS Press; 2004.
15. Ganapathy K. Telemedicine in India. Asia Pacific Biotech News 10:15. 2006. http://www.asiabiotech.com/readmore/vol10/1019/telemed.html.
16. Ganapathy K. Telehealth: yesterday, today and tomorrow. *Computer Soc India Commun.* 2007;30(11):5-11.
17. Ganapathy K, Ravindra A. *Telemedicine in Neurosciences in Current Principles and Practice of Telemedicine and e-Health.* Amsterdam: IOS Press; 2008:149-169.
18. Ganapathy K, Ravindra A. Healthcare for rural India: is telemedicine the solution? *J E Health Technol Appl.* 2007;5:203-207.
19. Ganapathy K, Ravindra A. mHealth: a potential tool for health care delivery in India. 2008. Available at: http://www.ehealth-connection.org/files/conf-materials/mHealth_A%20potential%20tool%20in%20India_0.pdf.
20. Grady JL, Schlachta-Fairchild L. International telenursing survey. *Comput Inform Nurs.* 2007;25:266-272.
21. Guilfoyle C, Perry L, Lord B, et al. Developing a protocol for the use of telenursing in community health in Australia. *J Telemed Telecare.* 2002;8:33-36.
22. Hagan L, Morin D, Lépine R. Evaluation of telenursing outcomes: satisfaction, self-care practices, and cost savings. *Public Health Nurs.* 2000;17:305-313.
23. Hardin S, Langford D. Telehealth's impact on nursing and the development of the interstate compact. *J Prof Nurs.* 2001;17:243-247.
24. Hartford K. Telenursing and patients' recovery from bypass surgery. *J Adv Nurs.* 2005;50:459-468.
25. Henderson K. TelEmergency: distance emergency care in rural emergency departments using nurse practitioners. *J Emerg Nurs.* 2006;32:388-393.
26. Hibbert D, Mair FS, Angus RM, et al. Lessons from the implementation of a home telecare service. *J Telemed Telecare.* 2003;9:55-56.

27. Holmström I. Decision aid software programs in telenursing: not used as intended? Experiences of Swedish telenurses. *Nurs Health Sci.* 2007;9:23-28.
28. Holmström I, Höglund AT. The faceless encounter: ethical dilemmas in telephone nursing. *J Clin Nurs.* 2007;16:1865-1871.
29. http://mohfw.nic.in/NRHM/asha.htm.
30. http://www.domain-b.com/industry/telecom/20090221_indias_phone_connections.html.
31. http://www.hindu.com/2008/01/22/stories/2008012250520200.htm.
32. http://www.ihe-online.com/index.php?id=2695.
33. http://www.indiannursingcouncil.org/pdf/statistics-2006.pdf.
34. http://www.isft.net/cms/index.php?telenursing.
35. http://www.rediff.com/money/2007/apr/30school.htm.
36. http://www.rediff.com///news/2006/jul/05spec.htm.
37. http://www.trai.gov.in/WriteReadData/trai/upload/StudyPapers/12/studypaper16dec08.pdf.
38. Atlas: Nurses in Mental Health 2007 (2007) © World Health Organization
39. Jerant AF, Azari R, Martinez C, et al. A randomized trial of telenursing to reduce hospitalization for heart failure: patient-centered outcomes and nursing indicators. *Home Health Care Serv Q.* 2003;22:1-20.
40. Johnston B, Heeler J, Dueser K, et al. Outcomes of the Kaiser Permante tele-home health research project. *Arch Fam Med.* 2000;9:40-45. http://telemedtoday.com/articlearchive/articles/Tele-homeHealthII.htm.
41. Kaminsky E, Rosenqvist U, Holmström I. Telenurses' understanding of work: detective or educator? *J Adv Nurs.* 2009;65(2):382-390.
42. Kawaguchi T, Azuma M, Ohta K. Development of a telenursing system for patients with chronic conditions. *J Telemed Telecare.* 2004;10:239-244.
43. Kim HS, Kim NC, Ahn SH. Impact of a nurse short message service intervention for patients with diabetes. *J Nurs Care Qual.* 2006;21:266-271.
44. Larsen BS, Clemensen J, Ejskjaer N. A feasibility study of UMTS mobile phones for supporting nurses doing home visits to patients with diabetic foot ulcers. *J Telemed Telecare.* 2006;12:358-362.
45. Leclerc BS, Dunnigan L, Côté H, et al. Callers' ability to understand advice received from a telephone health-line service: comparison of self-reported and registered data. *Health Serv Res.* 2003;38:697-710.
46. Lillibridge J, Hanna B. Using telehealth to deliver nursing case management services to HIV/AIDS clients. *Online J Issues Nurs.* 2009;14(1):36-40.
47. Lorentz MM. Telenursing and home healthcare. The many facets technology. *Home Healthc Nurse.* 2008;26:237-243.
48. McDermott R. Telenursing can reduce costs and improve access for rural patients. *Oncol Nurs Forum.* 2005;32:16.
49. Paul PG, Raman R, Rani PK, et al. Patient satisfaction levels during teleophthalmology consultation in rural South India. *Telemed J E Health.* 2006;12:571-578.
50. Peck A. Changing the face of standard nursing practice through telehealth and telenursing. *Nurs Adm Q.* 2005;29:339-343.
51. Roberts D, Tayler C, MacCormack D, et al. Telenursing in hospice palliative care. *Can Nurse.* 2007;103:24-27.
52. Rosina R, Starling J, Nunn K, et al. Telenursing: clinical nurse consultancy for rural paediatric nurses. *J Telemed Telecare.* 2002;8:48-49.
53. Russo H. Window of opportunity for home care nurses: telehealth technologies. *Online J Issues Nurs.* 2001;6:4. http://www.nursingworld.org/ojin/topic16/tpc16_4.htm
54. Scalvini S, Martinelli G, Baratti D, et al. Telecardiology: one-lead electrocardiogram monitoring and nurse triage in chronic heart failure. *J Telemed Telecare.* 2005;11:18-20.

55. Scalvini S, Volterrani M, Giordano A, et al. Boario home care project: an Italian telemedicine experience. *Monaldi Arch Chest Dis.* 2003;60:254-257.
56. Schlachta-Fairchild L. Telehealth: a new venue for health care delivery. *Semin Oncol Nurs.* 2001;17:34-40.
57. Snooks HA, Williams AM, Griffiths LJ, et al. Real nursing? The development of telenursing. *J Adv Nurs.* 2008;61:631-640.
58. St George I, Cullen M, Gardiner L, et al. Universal telenursing triage in Australia and New Zealand – a new primary health service. *Aust Fam Physician.* 2008;37:476-479.
59. Tschirch P, Walker G, Calvacca LT. Nursing in tele-mental health. *J Psychosoc Nurs Ment Health Serv.* 2006;44:20-27.
60. Vincent C, Reinharz D, Deaudelin I, et al. Public telesurveillance service for frail elderly living at home, outcomes and cost evolution: a quasi experimental design with two follow-ups. *Health Qual Life Outcomes.* 2006;4:41.
61. Vitacca M, Assoni G, Pizzocaro P, et al. A pilot study of nurse-led, home monitoring for patients with chronic respiratory failure and with mechanical ventilation assistance. *J Telemed Telecare.* 2006;12(7):337-342.
62. Wootton R, Loane M, Mair F, et al. The potential for telemedicine in home nursing. *J Telemed Telecare.* 1998;4:214-218.
63. Yun EK, Park HA. Factors affecting the implementation of telenursing in Korea. *Stud Health Technol Inform.* 2006;122:657-659.
64. Yun EK, Park HA. Strategy development for the implementation of telenursing in Korea. *Comput Inform Nurs.* 2007;25:301-306.

Telenursing in Chronic Conditions

6

Takayasu Kawaguchi, Masumi Azuma, Masae Satoh, and Yoji Yoshioka

Abbreviations

ANA	American Nurses Association
BMI	Body Mass Index
CBT	Cognitive Behavioral Therapy
CNAS	College of Nursing Art and Science, Hyogo, JAPAN
e-Japan	Electronic-Japan Strategy
e-mail	Electronic-mail
ICT	Information and Communications Technology
IT	Information Technology
PC	Personal Computer
PHS	Personal Handy-phone System
THA	Total Hip Arthroplasty
WHO	World Health Organization

6.1
Background/Setting

6.1.1
Setting/Brief Description of Health-care System

Advances in computer science and information technology (IT) are giving rise to the rapid development of health-care databases and related information systems. The health-care environment is undergoing rapid changes as information systems develop. Disease structure is also changing, from being dominated by acute and chronic infectious diseases to

T. Kawaguchi (✉)
Doctoral Program in Nursing Sciences, Graduate School of Comprehensive Human Sciences, University of Tsukuba, Tennodai, Tsukuba, Ibaraki, 305-8577, Japan
e-mail: kawat@md.tsukuba.ac.jp

S. Kumar and H. Snooks (eds.), *Telenursing*, Health Informatics,
DOI: 10.1007/978-0-85729-529-3_6, © Springer-Verlag London Limited 2011

being dominated by lifestyle-related diseases. As the size of the elderly population increases, this change in disease structure is becoming more pronounced. Periods of illness are becoming longer, and an increasing number of people have illnesses or disorders. There are an increasing number of cases in which patients undergo treatment as they go about their regular lives in the community and family. The World Health Organization (WHO) announced that an increasing number of people are suffering from chronic diseases worldwide, such as heart disease, stroke, cancer, and diabetes. These disorders will claim the lives of an estimated 35 million people in 2005, representing 60% of all deaths. In such situations, patient health-care needs become more diverse and there is a demand for high-quality health-care services that offer the types and levels of service that can be tailored to meet the needs of individuals.

As these changes occur, attention is turning to telenursing as a new means of providing continuous nursing care for patients with lifestyle-related and other chronic diseases. Chronic diseases often found in the recipients of at-home care services are listed below.[27] Patients with these chronic diseases can receive telenursing care.[4,7,9,10,12,14,16,18,19,24,30]

1. Diabetes
2. Hypertension
3. Congestive heart failure
4. Coronary artery disease
5. Chronic obstructive pulmonary disease
6. Cancer
7. Degenerative neurologic disorders
8. AIDS

The American Nurses Association (ANA) defines telenursing as "a form of telehealth where the focus is on nursing practice via telecommunications."[1,2] It is defined as the nursing practice in which two-way telecommunications are used for nurse and patient interactions to obtain information showing the patient's state of health and provide care and patient education through medical interventions and treatments.[5] Implementating telenursing requires that health and lifestyle information be obtained from distant sites and that client nursing information be understood comprehensively.

For example, in chronic diseases such as diabetes mellitus there is a strong relationship between overeating and lack of exercise, obesity, and psychological and social stress; such diseases are caused by living habits that are difficult to alter. Diabetes treatments are centered on dietary, exercise, and drug therapies, and patients themselves must incorporate lifelong treatment methods into their daily lives, managing themselves while living with the disease. In such diseases that require self-management over long periods, actual self-management behaviors are difficult to maintain, even if the patient has strong intentions to carry them out, and complications occur in many cases. Therefore, mental support for the family and expert, and continuous support from medical professionals are needed in patient treatment. In current medical practice, however, involvement is limited to short-term hospitalization for patient education and outpatient visits once every 2–3 months. Continuous support matching patient lifestyle is very difficult. In this chapter, we describe efforts to develop a practical telenursing support system that is being implemented with the aim of providing professional support to patients with chronic disease who are leading normal lives in society while undergoing treatment at home.[8]

6.1.2
Nursing Practice in the Country

In Japan, with the aging of society, the importance of continuous nursing care for chronically ill patients keeps increasing. Against this background, telenursing shows promise as an important means of nursing care in the future. However, a number of significant issues must be addressed before telenursing can be properly implemented. The first problem is "information literacy." In other words, individuals who receive nursing care do not have sufficient knowledge of using IT devices. In addition, although the development of IT devices is making rapid progress, difficulty in operating these devices is also a challenging issue while such devices remain in the developmental phase.

The second problem is the lack of establishment of sufficient infrastructure. Information and communications technology (ICT) is rapidly advancing, but the hardware, such as for optical communication, which is necessary to implement telenursing, is not available in all regions of Japan. Telenursing can be particularly effective in depopulated areas, but infrastructure delays in these regions remain problematic.

The third problem is a delay in legal frameworks concerning "protection of personal information." The security necessary for personal information flow over the Internet has not been completely ensured. In addition, the legal rules applicable to an information society have not been fully discussed. This has given rise to frequent criminal activity.

6.1.3
Telecommunications and Other Relevant Infrastructure/Resource Information

The e-Japan strategy office was established in Japan's Cabinet Office in January 2001 amidst global trends toward computerization, and full-scale infrastructure development began (http://www.kantei.go.jp/foreign/policy/it/index_e.html).[25] In the same year, a basic IT law was established and Japan made its first real efforts toward becoming the world's leading IT nation. As a result, basic infrastructure was rapidly developed by 2003, and in that year more than half of the Japanese population had access to the Internet. In 2003, efforts started with a focus on seven leading areas with the aim of more specific development: medical care, food, daily living, small business financing, knowledge, employment and labor, and government services. In 2004, investigations were begun on assessment methods and regulatory reforms for international strategies. Telemedicine and telenursing was considered to be one of the most important measures in the seven leading fields, and development of various types of software was started in the private sector. As this infrastructure was rapidly developed, important issues and problems that needed to be dealt with were noted. These included security problems, delayed development of social systems to make these other systems practical, and the problem of IT literacy among users. To deal with these issues, quick progress was made

in the development of the legal environment in Japan, while at the same time, IT education was made compulsory in school curricula, from the elementary and middle school
levels to university education.

Increasing Internet use is growing globally, and forms of communication are changing
at a fast pace. Under these circumstances, the acronym ICT is coming into more general
use than IT today. The USA has an advanced form of ICT, and one in ten American Internet
users is aged 50 years or older. Some 60% of these are thought to use medical, health, and
welfare consultations sites. This trend is also known as "e-health" or "e-hospitals," and
there are great expectations for a shift in economic circles to something that will have a
large impact on the senior market in the twenty-first century. Five characteristics may be
given for the information services provided by e-health: (1) content (the latest, updated
information and knowledge is available), (2) connectivity (easy access is possible without
regard to place or time), (3) community (groups of people with the same interests can be
formed), (4) commerce (these systems can function to mediate various business dealings),
and (5) e-health (medicine, medical care, health, and welfare information services can be
received). The roles needed to fulfill these service functions are thought to provide an
opportunity to transform the paradigms in the medical care, health, and welfare fields in
moving toward patient-centered medicine.[3]

6.1.4
General Background on Telehealth/Telemedicine in the Country

As we move toward rapidly evolving e-health and e-hospitals, telenursing will probably play
an important role as care expands through ICT. Serious diseases that need to be dealt with in
developed countries with aged populations include cancer, dementia, neurological and psychiatric disorders, and lifestyle-related diseases including diabetes, hyperlipidemia, hypertension, arteriosclerosis, and motor disorders of the bone and muscle. A characteristic of these
diseases is that support is required not only for the person suffering from the disease, but also
for the people providing care. In Japan, however, little attention is given to the activities of
people providing this type of care; support systems extend only to medical institutions whose
activities are covered under national health-care insurance and such activities do not function
as professional care. In such situations, Japan lags furthest behind among the developed countries, and urgent measures including reform of the medical service fee system are needed.

6.2
Current Telenursing Practice

6.2.1
General Statistics: Extent of Telenursing/Number of Programs

According to the "Report of the 2004–2005 International Telenursing Survey," using
telenursing can greatly expand the field of activity of nurses.[11] However, many issues must
be resolved to implement telenursing. These issues include compensation in case of acci-

dents, establishment and responsibility for certification systems, maintenance of strict confidentiality, and ensuring quality of care.

Amidst the urgency to resolve such issues, telenurses around the world who are actually engaged in telenursing are doing so on a part-time basis; the proportion is about 50%. The most frequent work sites are hospitals (27.0%), followed by colleges (11.0%), communities (9.7%), call centers (8.9%), and the governmental organizations (8.2%).

The annual salary for telenursing in the USA ranges from $50,000 to $75,000, and the annual salary worldwide (US dollar-equivalent) ranges from $35,000 to $75,000. The types of care provided by telenurses, in order of descending frequency, are chronic care, basic medical–surgical care, pediatric care, coronary care, psychiatric care, obstetric care, orthopedic care, neurological care, neonatal care, and rehabilitative care. As utilization increases, areas in which there is an urgent need for research and development include using of remote monitoring devices, handheld and mobile computers, and robots. Areas in which utilization is expected to decrease include telehealth tools, telephone-only interaction, online consumer health, and decision support tools. However, in telenursing, planning educational curriculum, establishing a certification system, and ensuring adequate personnel are priority targets.

6.2.2
Policy and Operational Challenges

Advanced ICT countries, such as the USA and the UK, are leading efforts for practical systems of telenursing.[20,26,31] In Japan, however, the ground has not been sufficiently prepared to take in these efforts. Differences in communication circumstances, health-care environments, and culture also make it difficult in various aspects to immediately accept unconditionally and keep up with the movements in those advanced countries. In the actual operation of telenursing in Japan, original system structure processes based on current medical environments, culture, and climate are needed. In Japan, moving toward ICT is a key policy promoted by the national government, and efforts to move toward practical telenursing with reforms in the health, medical, and welfare systems to match the advances in ITC have finally begun to attract attention.

In Japan, preparations are being made for all-digital domestic broadcasts, with a targeted date of July 2011, as one stage of infrastructure completion. Television broadcasts permeate daily life, and with their digitalization the Internet penetration rate is expected to explode. Telenursing systems via television have thus begun to be investigated. A preparatory stage for that is the appearance of a new academic discipline called nursing informatics in the field of nursing. In the USA and other countries, clinical nurse specialists who have mastered nursing IT are registered, and there are many settings in which they make use of that specialization. In Japan, a similar qualification system is now being considered. The essential features of such a course are mastering certain skills in nursing science, IT, and computer science. There is currently only one educational institution in Japan where this can be studied, the nursing information science course in the Graduate School of Applied Informatics, University of Hyogo. Issues requiring urgent attention are establishment of a qualification system, increasing the number of educational institutions that provide such courses, and training specialists who can handle telenursing professionally as an effective means of care.

6.2.3
Specific Program Examples/Best Practices

Continuous nursing care using telenursing will be an important step in the provision of care for patients with chronic conditions who need long-term follow-up care. Following are two examples from Japan of attempts at continuous nursing care for patients with chronic diseases using telenursing.

6.2.3.1
Telenursing for Type 2 Diabetes Patients

The effort described here is a telenursing support system based on mobile computing for home treatment of patients with chronic disease.[13] Telenursing is provided via the Internet for patients, particularly those with chronic diseases, who are self-managing their healthcare, while periodically visiting hospitals as outpatients. An outline of the system is shown in Fig. 6.1. It consists of a network in which there is interaction through a CNAS healthcare center between nurses at several subcenters located in a given region, patients under the management of the subcenter, and their attending physicians. A database server located at a university regional care center functions as the main database facility, and patients, nurses, and doctors input and view necessary information via a website. Currently, security is assured with the use of personal ID. The system also incorporates data mining and data

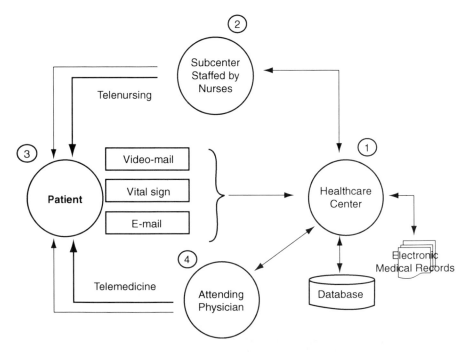

Fig. 6.1 Next-generation telenursing support system (Adapted from Okawa et al.[24])

warehouse functions so that it can quickly find and present necessary information or targeted information from vast amounts of data. The subcenters are staffed by specialist nurses, knowledgeable about information and telecommunications, who visit multiple patients in the target region and directly perform nursing tasks.

Three types of information from patients that is needed in providing telenursing care are used in this system. The first is written e-mail exchanges with daily consultations. The second is vital sign e-mails in which vital indicators such as blood pressure, temperature, and polls are regularly measured and sent. The third type is video-mail with actual health consultations through video images.[22,23] The patients themselves input these different types of information daily, and the following day the nurse in charge collects this information through the regional care center and decides, depending on the received data, whether to provide care via telenursing communication or to visit the patient personally. The system is also devised so that information can be shared with the attending physician in cases when medical procedures are necessary.

Figure 6.1 shows the system constructed to provide this kind of telenursing. The patients, subcenter nurses, and attending physicians always carry mobile PCs wherever they go to communicate wirelessly (128 Kbps) with the use of PHS cards. The system is set up so that patients can access the database server via the Internet, send files, or view their own daily health status on the website.

A trial using this system was conducted for 5 months with a male patient with type 2 diabetes, and significant improvements ($P<0.001$) were seen in blood sugar, HbA1c, and blood pressure levels. The patient who used the system was also very satisfied, and it led to good results in self-care. However, the nurses providing the care said that hardware operation placed considerable burdens on their time, which suggests that a number of issues remain to be addressed in using mobile computers in telenursing.

6.2.3.2
Telenursing for a Patient Following Total Hip Arthroplasty

Here, we introduce an example of a telenursing program developed to provide continuous nursing for a patient who had undergone total hip arthroplasty (THA), as a key element in the telenursing support system. Following THA there are risks of dislocation, wear, or infection of the artificial joint that can lead to the need for a second replacement operation. In particular, dislocation and wear are easily affected by a (home) lifestyle where, for example, floor chairs or cushions are regularly used, as in Japan. THA patients need continuous nursing throughout life.

An outline of this telenursing support program is shown in Fig. 6.2. This program is broadly divided into (1) general support from evidence based on existing knowledge and experience and (2) individual support using assessment and educational tools. For general support, information that needs to be shared with the patient is provided. For individual support, patient conditions are assessed objectively and subjectively using independently disease-specific scales that have been developed. The system is devised to provide more specific educational and nursing support needed by individuals classified by type. The experiences of experts are reflected in these assessment and educational support contents.

Data exchanged with patients through this telenursing support program are collected in the database, and finally fed back to the telenursing support system through data mining and data warehouses. This data also help to assure the quality of subsequent nursing support.

In order to provide follow-up guidance (but not initial guidance) on the management of metabolic syndrome, the Ministry of Health, Labour and Welfare has approved the use of information and communications equipment since April 2008, with the aim of reducing medical expenditure. Thus, the practice of telenursing in Japan is expected to grow even more in the future.

6.2.4
Information on Outcomes/Impact of Telenursing Programs (Preferably Quantitative and Not Anecdotal)

Patient education is essential in the care of chronic diseases. Here, we introduce research that systematically reviews the effectiveness of patient education using a computer communication network, comprising Internet websites, e-mail, bulletin boards, and charts.

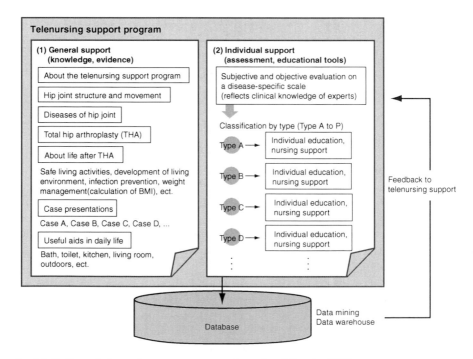

Fig. 6.2 Outline of telenursing support program for patient following THA

First, we discuss a study on patient education using a website. In a study on patients with depression, Christensen et al.[6] used a website with cognitive behavioral therapy (CBT) to prevent depression for intervention group 1, and a website providing information, together with treatment for intervention group 2. In a control group, the interviewer made phone calls. The results showed that in intervention groups 1 and 2, knowledge of CBT increased and depression improved compared to the control group.

Kukafka et al.[15] compared and evaluated the effects of a system using a website for self-efficacy in patients with acute myocardial infarction. In intervention group 1, a model tailored to patient characteristics was shown. In intervention group 2, a general website was used. In the control group, pamphlets were used. An intergroup comparison was not conducted, but in intervention group 1, the results showed a significant difference between before and after 1 month in terms of behavior and awareness, and between before and after 3 months in terms of behavior, awareness, and symptoms. In intervention group 2, *no* significant differences were noted.

Next, in a study of patient education using a website and e-mail, Strom et al.[29] provided feedback by e-mail in response to reports like sleep diaries from patients with insomnia via a website. With regard to total awake time, total sleep time, and sleep efficiency, significant main effects and interactions were seen in the intervention group.

In a study by Oenema et al.,[21] an intervention group received knowledge about nutrition and offered a nutrition diagnosis program on a website. The group input information and received individual feedback on nutritional status. In a control group, a letter on the importance of a healthy diet, the present state of national nutrition, and recipes for a low-fat diet were provided. In parameters such as the intention to reduce fat intake, results showed a significant effect in the intervention group compared to the control group.

In another study of patient education using a website and bulletin board, Lorig et al.[17] conducted a single e-mail discussion group for several days as intervention among patients with chronic back pain. In addition to conventional care, a control group received a subscription to a non-health-related magazine. Results for the intervention group showed significant improvement in health-related items, without any significant difference in health-care utilization.

Southard et al.[28] conducted patient education using a website, e-mail, and a bulletin board in patients diagnosed with coronary artery disease, congestive heart failure, or both. The intervention group accessed a website that provided information and input data. They could also participate in an online discussion group and link to related sites. The control group received conventional care. Weight and BMI (body mass index) were significantly lower in the intervention group than in the control group, but no significant differences were seen in other parameters.

Studies to date have reported that intervention using websites and e-mail is more effective than other types of intervention. In other words, this suggests that two-way interactive communication is more effective than one-way information via a website for patient education. Furthermore, even when intervention via a bulletin board was added, no big improvement in result was noted. Thus, even with interactive messages, a message from a specific person is educationally more effective.

6.3
Future Directions

6.3.1
Program Expansion

Computerization in hospitals and other facilities is rapidly developing as information-based societies continue to evolve. However, computerization of medicine and nursing in rural areas is lagging. For telenursing to function as a means to keep up with information-based societies, efforts will be needed to match the characteristics of local health care.

In an advanced, information ubiquitous society (information-based society in which necessary information can be obtained anytime, anywhere), systematization of telenursing so that it meets social needs will be looked to more and more as new needs appear. This will require investigation of telenursing methods to create a local care environment in which care can be provided with assurance, the creation of government systems to realize this and the creation of systems to provide related information. In development to build telenursing information networks that correspond to local health-care systems, it is important to match the system to the characteristics of the local health-care community. For example, in health-care communities that are trying to enhance high-level health-care services, advancing the systematization of hospital medical care and medical care provision systems and establishing systems that connect health, medicine, and welfare are necessary. In communities that are trying to focus on primary care that is close to the lives of community residents, health-care systems need to be developed that are suited to the health needs of the people living in those communities.

For these systems to link organically in community medical care and function effectively as networks, it is also important to build information sharing systems of local medical care between health-care communities. In other words, the nurse in charge and primary care physician serve important roles, being responsible for the patient's and his or her family's health information, including daily health management and prevention of lifestyle-related disease, providing comprehensive medical care, and promoting coordination of care efforts. The creation of suitable information systems is also needed to share information between nurses in charge, primary care physicians, and central hospitals in the community; coordinating and setting up relevant departments; using medical facilities jointly, supporting the establishment of open hospital beds; creating systems to promote coordinated care and referring patients; developing reverse referral systems; and providing and supporting professional knowledge.

Increases in bedridden patients or those with intractable diseases are predicted as society ages, and there is an increasing need for the provision of appropriate medical care in the home and medical care that aims to improve patient quality of life, while respecting their desire to be treated at home. In the future, there is expected to be an increasing need for the development of telemedicine and telenursing, together with conventional visiting medical care and visiting nursing. Moreover, in building these systems, development with a view toward smooth use and management of information during emergencies or disasters; coordination of information with care insurance service providers, volunteers, or other parties; comprehensive consultations; and creation of service provision systems is also necessary.

6.3.2
Policy

As the information society continues to develop, telenursing is a promising novel approach to medical and nursing care. In Europe and the USA, along with advances in IT, e-health is evolving and has been effective in applications such as home health care involving outpatient nursing and chronically ill patients. The way in which e-health is evolving in the USA, England, and Northern Europe differs depending on private or government initiatives, but results are being achieved in relation to seeking solutions to deal with health care and elderly care problems, which are common in all developed countries. However, in the USA, telemedicine and telenursing, because of implementation by private medical management companies, are being influenced by the management practices and policies of those companies, and many inadequacies remain in providing continued high-quality telemedical and telenursing care. Even in the USA, as policy measures at the national and state government level, a legal framework (including assistance and regulations) is necessary.

On the other hand, in Japan, despite rapid advances in ICT, the spread of telemedicine and telenursing relatively still lags. University research facilities and private medical organizations have made efforts in some municipalities, and at the national level, an examination of approaches is proceeding at a rapid pace. To date, one of the factors impeding the spread of telenursing in Japan has been problems with health insurance and medical fee reimbursement systems. Telenursing is not covered by health insurance, thus offering no economic incentives for telenursing. The same is true for the nursing-care insurance system in Japan. Nursing care provided remotely to homes is not covered for reimbursement. If medical and nursing care via telecommunication were covered by insurance, the technologies would be more widely adopted. To achieve this, policy measures must be taken to revise the health insurance system and reform medical and nursing reimbursement. In addition, teleservices require more advanced imaging, so establishing the infrastructure for telecommunication is important. To promote this infrastructure and deal with high transmission costs, policy measures must also be taken for additional items such as connection fees and maintenance costs.

Practical use of telenursing technology has four requirements: implementation, research, education, and management. To expand telenursing services in Japan, government and administrative policy measures concerning these four requirements are necessary. To facilitate practical operation, government and administrative authorities must take the lead and, as policy tasks, must make policy decisions and appropriate budgets, and move toward implementing specific policies, including starting model programs in local municipalities and designing subsidy systems. To promote administrative policy decisions, scientific data are needed as a basis for assessing the effectiveness of telenursing. Doing so requires practical research results from universities, research facilities, and medical care organizations. Policy assistance like support for such research is also necessary. In addition, telenursing is a new service technology, so educational systems must be established to teach telenursing and provide necessary academic resources, including training of new personnel in nursing informatics. This educational framework also demands policy action. Furthermore, information and communication involve ethical issues such as privacy protection. This also requires administrative policy, including a legal framework.

Issues of medical care and medical costs faced by Japan and foreign countries in dealing with their aging societies will continue to grow in the future. Telemedicine and telenursing, as a solution for these issues, are effective methods. Expansion and promotion of this technology is, in a certain sense, the missions for the government and health-care professionals. To achieve a society in which everyone can receive appropriate services, "whenever, wherever, and whoever" needs it, government, medical organizations, and university research and educational institutions must unite efforts toward expanding telenursing services. This is true not only for Japan, but for developed countries as well.

6.4
Summary

- Telenursing is a new means of providing continuous nursing care for patients with lifestyle-related and other chronic diseases.
- As we move toward rapidly evolving e-health and e-hospitals, telenursing is likely to play an important role as care expands through ICT.
- Issues requiring urgent attention are establishment of a qualification system, increasing the number of educational institutions that provide such courses and training specialists who can handle telenursing professionally as an effective means of care.
- Continuous nursing with the use of telenursing will be an important step in the provision of care for chronic disease patients who need long-term follow-up care.
- Two examples of attempts at continuous nursing for patients with chronic diseases using telenursing in Japan are: (1) telenursing for type 2 diabetes patients and (2) telenursing for a patient following THA.
- In order to develop telenursing information networks that correspond to local health-care systems, it is important to match the system to the characteristics of the local health-care community.
- In the future, there is expected to be an increasing need for the development of telemedicine and telenursing, together with conventional visits from medical care and visiting nurses.
- In building these systems, development with a view toward smooth use and management of information during emergencies or disasters, coordination of information with care insurance service providers, volunteers or other parties, comprehensive consultations, and creation of service provision systems are also necessary.

Acknowledgments We are thankful to our supervisor, Kenichi Ohta, whose encouragement, guidance, and support from the initial to the final level enabled us to develop an understanding of the subject. Finally, we are also grateful to all who supported us in any way during the completion of the project.

Glossary

Chronic conditions – Have persistent or recurring health consequences lasting for years. They are illnesses or impairments that cannot be cured. Some of the most prevalent chronic conditions, such as sinusitis or hay fever, are generally not disabling; however, others, such as heart disease and arthritis, can cause significant limitations in people's ability to perform certain basic activities of daily living (ADLs). Thus, in addition to medical services, people who have chronic conditions often need personal, social, or rehabilitative care over a prolonged period of time. *Source*: National Academy on an Aging Society (homepage on the Internet). Washington: The Academy; c1999–2009. Chronic conditions: A challenge for the twenty-first century. 1999; 1, November: 2. Available from http://hpi.georgetown. edu/agingsociety/pdfs/chronic.pdf (cited 9 March 2010).

Chronic diseases – Are non-communicable illnesses that are prolonged in duration, do not resolve spontaneously, and are rarely cured completely. Examples of chronic diseases include heart disease, cancer, stroke, diabetes, and arthritis. *Source*: Centers for Disease Control and Prevention (homepage on the Internet). Atlanta: The Centers; c1946–2009. Chronic disease prevention and health promotion: What are chronic diseases? Available from http://www.cdc.gov/nccdphp/publications/AAG/chronic.htm (updated 24 November 2008; cited 9 March 2009).

Lifestyle-related diseases – Is the disease group related to lifestyles such as a dietary habits and exercise habits, rest, smoking, and drinking.

e-health – Electronic-health it is a relatively recent term for health-care practice which is supported by electronic processes and communication

e-hospitals – Electronic-hospitals it brings learning opportunities to the reach of hospital patients

References

1. American Nurses Association. *Core Principles on Telehealth*. Washington, DC: American Nurses Publishing; 1999.
2. Association American Nurses. Telehealth: a tool for nursing practice. *Nurse Trends Issues*. 1997;2(4):1-2.
3. Brown G. Technology in nurse education: a communication teaching strategy. *ABNF J*. 1999; 10(1):9-13.
4. Caceres C, Gomez EJ, Garcia F, et al. An integral care telemedicine system for HIV/AIDS patients. *Int J Med Inform*. 2006;75:638-642.
5. Chaffee M. A telehealth odyssey. *Am J Nurs*. 1999;99(7):27-32.
6. Christensen H, Griffiths KM, Jorm AF. Delivering interventions for depression by using the internet: randomized controlled trial. *Br Med J*. 2004;328(7434):265-268.
7. Coughlin J, Pope J, Leedle B. Old age, new technology, and future innovations in disease management and home health care. *Home Health Care Manag Pract*. 2006;18:196-207.
8. Darkins AW, Cary MA. *Telemedicine and Telehealth*. New York: Springer; 2000.
9. Farmer A, Gibson OJ, Tarassenko L, et al. A systematic review of telemedicine interventions to support blood glucose self-monitoring in diabetes. *Diabet Med*. 2005;22:1372-1378.
10. Fetzer S. Telehealth monitoring: a new nursing tool. *Nurs News*. 2004;28(2):15.
11. Grady JL, Schlachta-Fairchild L. Report of the 2004–2005 international telenursing survey. *Comput Inform Nurs*. 2007;25(5):266-272.
12. Hee-Sung K. Impact of web-based nurse's education on glycosylated haemoglobin in type 2 diabetic patients. *J Clin Nurs*. 2007;16:1361-1366.

13. Kawaguchi T, Azuma M, Ohta K. Development of a telenursing system for patients with chronic conditions. *J Telemed Telecare*. 2004;10:239-244.
14. Kobb R, Chumbler N, Brennan D, et al. Home telehealth: mainstreaming what we do well. *Telemed J E Health*. 2008;14:977-981.
15. Kukafka R, Lussier YA, Eng P, et al. Web-based tailoring and its effect on self-efficacy: result from the MI-HEART randomized controlled trial. *AMIA Annual Symposium Proceedings*, 2002, San Antonio, 410-414.
16. Liddy C, Dusseault JJ, Dahrouge S, et al. Telehomecare for patients with multiple chronic illnesses: pilot study. *Can Fam Physician*. 2008;54(1):58-65.
17. Lorig KR, Laurent DD, Deyo RA, et al. Can a back pain e-mail discussion group improve health status and lower health care costs? A randomized study. *Arch Intern Med*. 2002;162(7):792-796.
18. Malacarne M, Gobbi G, Pizzinelli P, et al. A point-to-point simple telehealth application for cardiovascular prevention: the ESINO LARIO experience. Cardiovascular prevention at point of care. *Telemed J E Health*. 2009;15(1):80-86.
19. Moore R, Britton B, Chetney R. Wound care using interactive telehealth. *Home Health Care Manag Pract*. 2005;17:203-212.
20. National Council of State Boards of Nursing. Telenursing: the regulatory implications for multistate regulation. *Issues*. 1996;17(3):8-9.
21. Oenema A, Brug J, Lechner L. Web-based tailored nutrition education: results of a randomized controlled trial. *Health Educ Res*. 2001;16(6):647-660.
22. Ohta K, Hata Y, Kawaguchi T. Tele-nursing system and recognition of facial expressions. *Proceedings of Image and Vision Computing*, 2000:258-262.
23. Ohta K, Kizaki T, Kawaguchi T. Recognition of facial expressions and multimedia processing for tele-nursing system. *Proceedings of World Automation Congress Second International Forum on Multimedia and Image Processing*, Maui; 2000.
24. Okawa A, Umeda T, Fukuchi N, et al. Development of a telesupport system for cancer outpatients. *Kitasato Med J*. 2008;38:1-8.
25. Prime Minister's Official Residence [homepage on the Internet]. Tokyo: IT policy: The e-Japan strategy. Available at: http://www.kantei.go.jp/jp/it/network/dai1/0122summary_j.html [updated January 22, 2001; cited March 9, 2010].
26. Robbins KC. Telenursing: using technology to deliver health care. *ANNA J*. 1998;25(2):134.
27. Sharpe CC. *Telenursing: Nursing Practice in Cyberspace*. Westport: Auburn House; 2001.
28. Southard BH, Southard DR, Nuckolls J. Clinical trial of an internet-based case management system for secondary prevention of heart disease. *J Cardiopulm Rehabil*. 2003;23(5):341-348.
29. Strom L, Pettersson R, Andersson G. Internet-based treatment for insomnia: a controlled evaluation. *J Consult Clin Psychol*. 2004;72(1):113-120.
30. Verhoeven F, van Gemert-Pijnen L, Dijkstra K, et al. The contribution of teleconsultation and videoconferencing to diabetes care: a systematic literature review. *J Med Internet Res*. 2007;9(5):e37.
31. Wootton R, Loane M, Mair F, et al. A joint US–UK study of home telenursing. *J Telemed Telecare*. 1998;4(1):83-85.

Telenursing in Korea

7

Eun Kyoung Yun and Hyeoun-Ae Park

Abbreviations

GDP   Gross Domestic Product
IT   Information Technology
PDA   Personal Digital Assistant

7.1
Introduction

Development of science and information and telecommunications technology has gradually improved our quality of life. With the health service market being no exception, greater attention is being given to the application of information and communication technology by health-care providers aiming to provide more detailed, customized and personalized health-care services in an efficient and effective manner. One such method is telenursing, which refers to the use of telecommunication technology in nursing to enhance patient care.[7] Through this system, nurses monitor patients' data and analyze their condition, and then suggest nursing advice which will potentially enhance patients' ability to achieve and maintain their health and wellness.

The aim of this chapter is to survey the past and current status of telenursing in Korea, and provide the future vision for the provision of quality health service by nurses using information and communication technology.

E.K. Yun (✉)
College of Nursing Science, Kyung Hee University, 1 Hoegi dong, Dongdaemun-gu, Seoul, 130-701, South Korea
e-mail: ekyun@khu.ac.kr

S. Kumar and H. Snooks (eds.), *Telenursing*, Health Informatics,
DOI: 10.1007/978-0-85729-529-3_7, © Springer-Verlag London Limited 2011

7.2
Background Information

7.2.1
About Korea

The Republic of Korea covers an area of about 100,032 km². In 2010, Korea had a population of about 50 million, and the GDP was $20,265. The government reported a total of 20,833 health institutions, and a doctor-to-patient ratio of 1:630. The infant mortality was 4 per 1,000 live births, and life expectancy was 75.1 years for men and 82.3 years for women, respectively.

7.2.2
ICT in Health Services in Korea

In terms of information and communication technology, Korea is ranked as the world leader in availability of high-speed Internet services. Korea's Internet penetration rate passed the 70% mark as of 2010, with about 77.8% of people over the age of 4 years having online access.[8] The continuing developments in IT have initiated the broad implication of information and communication technology into health-care sectors.

7.3
Past and Present Telenursing in Korea

7.3.1
Nurses' Participation in Telemedicine

To understand the history of telenursing in Korea, it is helpful to briefly review how telemedicine has been implemented and developed in Korea. In 1988, the pilot telemedicine project between Seoul National University Hospital and Yonchen Community Health Centre was initiated.[22] Since then, various types of telemedicine projects have been implemented and tested in both public and private sectors. Between 1999 and 2001, the Korean government funded IT venture companies, which established many telemedicine businesses. However, most projects failed or did not produce satisfactory results.[10]

At the same time a process for development of a regulatory framework for the implementation and operation of telemedicine was established by the Korean government. In 2002, the first telemedicine medical law was passed, which certified telemedicine as a medical practice. In addition, the regulations covering telemedicine facilities and systems were issued in 2003. Telemedicine was reactivated among IT companies, universities, and competitive hospitals. Moreover, along with the computerization of health-care system and services, the outcome of those telemedicine projects has been improving with national task and support for ubiquitous computing.[22]

Nurses had an important role to play in the implementation and operation process in telemedicine services in Korea. Along with the introduction and development of telemedicine in the late 1980s, many nurses have participated in various telemedicine projects as model developers or service providers. At that time, the common type of telemedicine model including nurse as an active participant was performed using a computerized videoconference system between consultant (e.g., physician) and nurse. Initially, those interventions were conducted to deliver quality health-care services to those who are living in rural areas or islands, and others who do not have easy access to medical services. Members of the target group were people of low socioeconomic level, older than 65 years or suffering from chronic diseases needing repeat medication prescription (e.g., diabetes mellitus and hypertension).[4,5] Nurses had digital equipment for auscultation or visualization. They also had Internet access, which allowed them to assess patient symptoms. After the nurses assessed the patients, the teleconsultation system allowed real-time transmission of the patient data to the physician. It also helped the nurses to communicate with the physicians in remote areas for follow-up treatments. The nurses' participation in telemedicine projects are proliferated in specific medical areas. However, direct teleconsultation using real-time data transmission between patient and nurses has rarely been conducted. That is, the synchronized visible or audible telemonitoring or teleconsultation in telenursing service has seldom been utilized in Korea. This might be due to the current obstacles that exist in telenursing practice itself, rather than the technical feasibility.

7.3.2
Proliferation of Teleconsultation in Telenursing

Asynchronous consultation, which can be referred to as "store and forward consultation," has been increasingly used in telenursing in Korea. Through this kind of store and forward transmission method, the nurse could collect and analyze patients' data, including self-monitoring biological data, symptoms, activities, as well as emotional evaluation, and then provide them with nurses' opinion.

Consultation by telephone in telenursing has been used extensively. Telephone consultation research was initiated to deliver nursing advice to patients discharged from hospitals. In Korea, it has been identified that the target group of telephone consultation included post-chemotherapy patient,[15] psychiatric patients and family,[18] postpartum women[20,25], and mothers.[23] Currently, this telephone advice is being increasingly provided by nursing staff in hospitals in Korea, with the aim of increasing both quality of care and patient satisfaction.[1,13] Nurses identify patients' current status, trends, and the needs of the patients and then coordinate with all the other health professionals or staff within the hospital, in order to create a suitable and quality health service plan for the respective individual consumers. It seems that telephone consultation could have potential in improving the patient's adherence, reducing unnecessary admission by inappropriate care, and increasing customer loyalty toward the use of medical facilities. However, research focusing on the long-term effect has been limited in Korea.

Another method frequently used in telenursing in Korea is web-based intervention. Web-based intervention has an advantage of asynchronous communication that does not require the presence of two parties, nurse and patient, at the same time. In Korea, web-based telenursing usually combines online and offline interventions. Patient education was commonly given by the nurse prior to discharge from the hospital, and then patient was suggested to consult the websites. Nurses developed various websites where patients or family members may list their symptoms or questions, and nursing consultation is offered in these areas. Nurses monitor and analyze the patients' data or trends collected for a certain period of time. Therefore, nursing advice mainly covers nonemergency conditions. In Korea, effective telenursing consultation through the Internet has been well developed in caring for diabetic,[11,14] hemodialysis[2], or hypertension patients[26], as well as for mother with first baby.[12] Initially, web-based telenursing in Korea was used for clinical care purposes, but, increasingly, it is being used for education of caregivers[12,16] as well as healthy people. This can be found in the studies of aging and well-being programs,[9,21] health promotion programs for university students[19], and safety education for elementary students.[3,24]

Apart from telemedicine conducted in Korea, which focused on symptom management in patients diagnosed with specific medical diseases, it can be said that most telenursing projects had more emphasis on supportive care of patients as well as family members. In other words, regardless of the way telenursing is provided, most of the recommendations for the patients and their families are aimed at supporting or modifying their behavior and attitude. For example, several telenursing studies conducted in Korea demonstrated that the application of technology in nursing was effective and reliable for blood sugar control in diabetic patients,[11,14] adherence to breastfeeding for postpartum mothers,[20,25] self-care management for post-chemotherapy patients,[15] and increased knowledge or adjustment ability for dementia patient caregivers.[17]

The characteristics of teleconsultation in telenursing, designed and conducted by nurses or nursing organizations independently, can be summarized as follows: highlighted intervention using the Internet or telephone, focused self-management, and targeted toward ill or healthy people. Moreover, the indicators assessed most often in the evaluation of telenursing projects in Korea were the typical variables related to specific clinical conditions. Examples include comparison of level of knowledge, activities, and psychosocial–emotional status. Research on technical usability, acceptability, and long-term effectiveness from financial or social perspectives has been relatively limited.

7.3.3
Current Development

At present, the personal digital assistant (PDA)-based system accessible to the Internet is being used in the field of community nursing care. Nurses enter the patients' data (e.g., vital signs, medication, and intervention) and transfer the data to main server using the PDA. The system also allows nurses to figure out the standardized nurse practice protocol, and helps them to make nursing diagnosis and provide nursing practice.[6] That is one of the recent developments in data transfer method using wireless technology in telenursing projects in Korea. Advanced IT infrastructures and competencies have the potential to further improve the application and accessibility in telenursing.

7.4
Issues on Telenursing in Korea

There are some issues and concerns that should be considered in relation with operation of telenursing in Korea. These include telenursing professional's responsibilities and potential liabilities, patient privacy, security and confidentiality, standardized protocol guidelines, and funding police. Many of the issues are yet to be solved definitively, and these should be approached carefully.[27]

7.5
Education Opportunity

Education or counseling within telenursing has been conducted by nurses or nurse practitioners. Suitably trained nurses would make it more effective and efficient both technically and managerially. Effective use of telemedicine technology as a way of providing nursing demands more highly educated and qualified nurses such as nurse practitioners and nurse specialists. Although there are many certified nursing programs in Korea, formal education in telenursing has never been established.

Telenursing professionals require support for collecting and evaluating relevant and qualified clinical data, and storing and forwarding clinical data to data repositories and clinical specialists. Therefore, knowledge and experience in technical and clinical domains are needed for nurses to successfully coordinate and make decisions in various situations in telenursing operation. In addition, the competencies required in telenursing are knowledge of process quality management and data/information management skills.

The nurse prepared to take on roles in telenursing should be educated in nursing informatics. In 2005, the discipline of nursing informatics, as a formal education program, started at the graduate school of Seoul National University. The curriculum of nursing informatics includes: (1) the representation of nursing data, information, and knowledge; (2) information management; and (3) issues of hospital information and/or public health information. Recently, most graduate schools of nursing in Korea are providing a course of nursing informatics, hospital information systems, and public health information to master or doctoral students as an elective course. Nursing informatics is being included extensively even in the undergraduate curriculum among competitive universities. There is no formal telenursing education program in Korea. However, the concepts and practical application have been covered in nursing informatics courses.

Nurses in telenursing should be acquainted with information and communication technology and be able to use nursing knowledge in relation with patient data analysis and nursing consultation. At present, since the specialized telenursing education program is nonexistent, nursing practitioners would be considered for telenursing operation if they are educated and prepared to manage health information using telenursing technology. Nurse practitioners having been qualified and proved nationally in the fields of oncology, gerontology, psychology, pediatrics, and maternity can be consulted to fulfill patients' needs.

7.6
Future Direction

A variety of U-Health devices that incorporate advanced telecommunication technologies have recently been developed and introduced into the international market. In 2003, to keep the IT growth alive, the Korean Government suggested a new IT roadmap aimed at ushering in a "ubiquitous" society. Everything dubbed "ubiquitous" means an environment where people can enjoy access to high-speed networks and advanced communication services anywhere and anytime through a ubiquitous computing network. Furthermore, with these national and social attention and support, it is expected that more advanced telenursing research and projects will be actively expanded in the future.

Telenursing is not merely the application of a device into nursing domain using the most cutting-edge technology currently available. It is also not a service that is carried out only at a fixed point in time or intervals. Instead, it can be defined as a value-added health delivery system that is created by amalgamating nursing knowledge from nurse professionals with the most appropriate health devices, which is then distributed through current IT systems. It should incorporate advances in technology in order to maximize the efficiency, productivity, and cost-effectiveness of telenursing. Thus, in cooperation with all possible core assets, protocols and procedures have to be put in place in order to explicitly address the needs of the health-care providers and individual consumers while taking into account the overall health-care objectives of the government and general population.

The vision of telenursing in Korea is to utilize the vast knowledge and experiences inherently embedded within the various fields of nursing to prevent disease and promote wellness, and eventually empower people to take greater control over their own health and well-being. Telenursing in Korea will also foster participation of local communities and other health-care professionals to eventually develop and manage programs to meet the people's health-care requirements. To accomplish the above goals, partnerships and networking among health professionals, the roles of government, community, educational institutions, and the general public will be crucial.

7.7
Summary

- The broad implications of information and communication technology have been initiated into health-care sectors in Korea.
- Many telenursing projects in Korea have successfully been carried out with more emphasis on supportive care of patients as well as family members in various fields of nursing.
- The characteristics of teleconsultation in Korea can be summarized as follows: highlighted intervention using the Internet or telephone, focused self-management, and targeted toward ill or healthy people.

- Some legal and practical issues still exist in relation to implementation and operation of telenursing rather than technical feasibility in Korea.
- The vision of telenursing in Korea is to utilize the vast knowledge and experiences inherently embedded within the various fields of nursing to prevent disease and promote wellness, and eventually empower people to take greater control over their own health and well-being.

Glossary

ICT – Information and communication technology.

References

1. Cho HS. *The Effects of Psychosocial Rehabilitation Nursing Program for Chronic Mental Inpatients of Long-Term Psychiatric Hospital* [Unpublished doctoral dissertation]. Busan: Graduate School of Kosin University; 2004.
2. Chung HJ. Hemodialysis nursing education program using web-based learning system. *Nurs Tamgu.* 2000;9(1):146-166.
3. Chung ES, Jeong IS, Song MG. Development and effect analysis of web-based instruction program to prevent elementary school students from safety accidents. *J Korean Acad Nurs.* 2004;34(3):485-494.
4. http://voice.gangnam.go.kr/rsshtmllink.odc?userid=&i_did=8&categorycode=C01C03C07#titles0
5. http://www.dt.co.kr/contents.html?article_no=2005033002010151686001
6. http://www.zdnet.co.kr/ArticleView.asp?artice_id=20090322153505
7. International Council of Nurses. Telenursing. Available at: http://www.icn.ch/matters_telenursing.htm. Accessed March 28, 2010.
8. Internet Use Survey. Statistics at a glance. 2010. Available at: http://isis.nic.or.kr. Accessed November 30, 2010.
9. Jung YM. Development of a web-based senescence preparation education program for successful aging for middle-aged adults. *J Korean Acad Nurs.* 2008;38(6):831-842.
10. Kim IS. Applying telemedicine in nursing. *Korean J Nursi Query.* 2000;9(1):46-69.
11. Kim HS. Effects of web-based diabetic education in obese diabetic patients. *J Korean Acad Nurs.* 2005;35(5):924-930.
12. Kim JS. Development and evaluation of a web-based support program for the maternal role of primiparas. *J Korean Acad Nurs.* 2005;35(1):165-176.
13. Kim AS. *Effects of Individualized Education and Telephone Calls on Health Behavior and Nursing Service Satisfaction of Hypertension Patient in Ambulatory Setting* [Unpublished master dissertation]. Jeon-Ju: Graduate School of Chonbuk National University; 2004.
14. Kim HS, Kim SK. Effects of Internet-based diabetic education on plasma glucose and serum lipids in female type 2 diabetic patients. *Korean J Women Health Nurs.* 2004;10(4):311-317.
15. Kim AS, Lee ES, Kim SH. Effects of telephone intervention as supportive nursing on self-care practices and quality of life for gynecological cancer patients under chemotherapy. *J Korean Acad Nurs.* 2007;37(5):744-753.

16. Lee NY, Kim YH. Development and evaluation of an e-learning program for mothers of premature infants. *J Korean Acad Nurs*. 2008;38(1):152-160.
17. Lee HJ, Kim KR, Kim JS, et al. Effects of the problem-solving telephone counseling on caregiving appraisal and coping in family caregivers of the older adults with dementia. *J Korean Gerontol Sci*. 2004;24(1):21-36.
18. Lee KL, Yang S. Effects of telephone interview for chronic mentally ill persons on psychiatric symptoms and daily living activities. *J Korean Acad Psychiatr Ment Health Nurs*. 2006;15(4):482-490.
19. Park MH. Development and evaluation of online aging and health management education for undergraduate students. *J Korean Acad Nurs*. 2007;37(4):540-548.
20. Park SH, Koh HJ. Effect of breast-feeding education and follow-up care on the breast-feeding rate and the breast-feeding method-focused on home visit and phone counseling. *Korean J Women Health Nurs*. 2001;7(1):30-43.
21. Park JS, Kwon SM. Effect of an on-line health promotion program connected with a hospital health examination center on health promotion behavior and health status. *J Korean Acad Nurs*. 2008;38(3):393-402.
22. Ryu SW. *Telemedicine: Trends and Issues*. Seoul: Korea Institute for Health and Social Welfare; 2002.
23. Song JH, Han KJ, Oh KS, et al. Analysis of telephone counseling service on child health. *Korean J Child Health Nurs*. 2001;7(2):245-257.
24. Song MG, Kim SJ. Development and effect analysis of web-based instruction program on safety for sixth grade elementary school students. *J Korean Acad Child Health Nurs*. 2006;12(2):233-243.
25. Yoo EK, Kim MH, Seo WS. A study on the rate of breast-feeding practice by education and continuous telephone follow-up. *Korean J Women Health Nurs*. 2002;8(3):424-434.
26. Yu JO, Cho YB. The effect of an Internet community on knowledge, self-efficacy and self care behavior in workers with hypertension. *J Korean Acad Nurs*. 2005;35(7):1258-1267.
27. Yun EK, Park HA. Strategy development for the implementation of telenursing in Korea. *Comput Inform Nurs*. 2007;25(5):301-306.

Telenursing in a Developing Country: The Philippine Experience

8

Joselito M. Montalban

Abbreviations

CHED   Commission on Higher Education
CHITS   Community Health Information Tracking System
ICT   Information and Communication Technology
ILHZ   Inter-local Health Zone
IT   Information Technology
NHIP   National Health Insurance Program
PGH   Philippine General Hospital
UP   University of the Philippines
VoIP   Voice-over Internet protocol
WWW   World Wide Web

Telenursing, the delivery of nursing services across a distance utilizing information and communication technology (ICT), is not yet a mainstream profession in the Philippines. Save for nurses taking part in an experimental or pilot telehealth project in a major university, it is unlikely that one would find a practicing nurse in the country list telenursing as an occupation or specialty. It is doubtful that even triage nurses in call centers run by managed care organizations would call themselves telenurses.

Nevertheless, if ICT were to be taken in its broad sense of computer-based information systems as well as any technology for transmitting, communicating, or broadcasting information, it can be argued that some form of telenursing has long been practiced in the country. The archipelagic nature of the country's geography with its 7,107 islands (see Fig. 8.1), coupled with a depleting health manpower resource, have compelled health-care providers to turn to ICT as a means for delivering some health, including nursing, services.

While the Internet is yet to make substantial inroads, especially in many remote and isolated communities, we can find short-wave radios and cellular phones extensively used by nurses in health centers and district hospitals dotting towns and villages, although these

J.M. Montalban
University of the Philippines in Manila, Cagayan de Oro, Philippines
e-mail: joselito.montalban@gmail.com

S. Kumar and H. Snooks (eds.), *Telenursing*, Health Informatics,
DOI: 10.1007/978-0-85729-529-3_8, © Springer-Verlag London Limited 2011

are used mainly for reporting accomplishment data for health statistics. Still, more advanced systems designed for the World Wide Web (WWW) and intended initially for use in select areas may eventually be extensively deployed nationwide. This will, of course, entail increased demand for a good number of nurses possessing relevant knowledge and skills in telehealth, and the country's educational sector should be able to meet this.

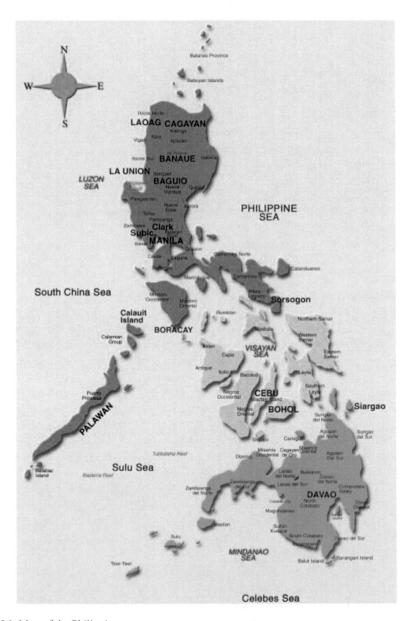

Fig. 8.1 Map of the Philippines

8.1
The Setting

By one estimate in 2006, 85% of nurses in the Philippines had left the country, with more expected to emigrate each year.[4] This trend is expected to persist through 2015. Already there is a shortage of nurses as well as doctors in hospitals and health centers. This is especially true in the countryside as many nurses opt for employment in regional and provincial hospitals in the cities where they can get better experience to improve chances of landing jobs abroad.[2] But even in these big hospitals, there is looming shortage. The Philippine General Hospital (PGH), which is the largest medical institution in the country, for example, loses 300–500 of its nurses each year,[1] although for the time being they are quickly replenished as work in this busy hospital is perceived as a valuable experience for employment abroad – so that nurses elsewhere in the country rush to fill vacancies created.

The foregoing scenario aggravates what is already an uneven distribution of health professionals in the country. A study commissioned by the International Labor Office in 2005 noted that most of them had been practicing in urban areas and only medical technologists, midwives, and barangay health workers had predominantly been located in rural areas.[5] The consequence of all these is an inequitable access to health care, with potential adverse impact on the health status of the country. This is a situation that is ripe for such innovations as telehealth.

Telehealth, or alternatively, telemedicine, which is a term often used synonymously, is defined as "the provision of health care services, clinical information, and education over a distance using telecommunication technology".[6] It is an emerging field that is seen to have great potential as supplementary means of delivering health services to remote communities where doctors, nurses, or other health professionals are either unavailable or lacking. It can be a way, therefore, to bridge the gap created by the prevailing situation of inequitable access to health care.

While there is no perfect substitute for face-to-face health care, telehealth is the best alternative if physically deploying health professionals is not feasible.

8.1.1
The Filipino Nurse in the District Health System

The district health system is defined by the World Health Organization as a more or less contained segment of the national health system. It comprises a well-defined administrative and geographic area, rural or urban, and includes all institutions and sectors contained in it whose activities contribute to improve health. It is applied primarily in countries like the Philippines where the responsibility of delivering health services has been transferred, or devolved, to local authorities. In line with this concept, in the Philippines, various health facilities are clustered into inter-local health zones (ILHZ), each of which has a defined population in a defined geographical area so that it is also called area health zone. These health facilities include a core referral hospital, which can be anything from a small community hospital to a large medical center and is the main point of referral for hospital services from the community and other health facilities within the area covered by the ILHZ.[3] In all of these health facilities, nurses play a crucial role as they are expected to be not only providers of care, but designers, managers, and coordinators of care as well. In this latter function, nurses serve as information managers, helping patients as well as other health professionals in their respective health facilities; outside their own health facilities, they acquire, interpret, and utilize information pertaining to promotive, preventive, curative, and rehabilitative care of the population, especially within the ILHZ. Thus, we see nurses perform tasks that fall within the purview of what has come to be known as telenursing, which is really a component of telehealth. These tasks may be anything from texting nursing advice through setting doctors' appointments over the telephone to reporting a town's infant mortality data to the provincial health office using a short-wave radio.

8.2
Initial Strides

The foregoing may as yet be what telenursing is mostly about in the Philippines. It is, by any measure, rudimentary, utilizing technologies such as telephone and radio, which, in today's high-tech digital world, may very well be classified as "old." Only recently has the use of computer systems and the WWW been explored. One landmark telemedicine initiative by a university is worth describing at some length.

8.2.1
BuddyWorks

The University of the Philippines' (UP) National Telehealth Center undertook a telemedicine project called "Design and Implementation of BuddyWorks: Using Telehealth Network Services in Community Partnership Project." It formally began on 1 January 2005. Planning and preparation took a good part of the first 2 years, with operations-proper commencing in January 2007.

The technology essentially consists of a web portal that handles digital images and text-based consults in store-and-forward or asynchronous mode. Through this portal and its short messaging system and voice-over internet protocol (VoIP) components, physicians and other health professionals in five hospitals, three medical schools, a provincial health office, and a municipal health office all over the country we are linked with specialists in the PGH, which is in the capital city of Manila (see Fig. 8.2), thus the moniker "BuddyWorks." As working buddies, they collaborated in improving health-care services through ICT.[7]

BuddyWorks provides a forum for doctors and other health professionals not only to send and receive referrals but also to confer and update their knowledge online (see Fig. 8.3). An interesting feature also is the web portal's telehealth nurse interface (see Fig. 8.4). This facilitates the system of sorting patients according to clinical needs called triaging. All referred cases are automatically populated on this page, where the telehealth nurses, or telenurses, can easily scan them and assign to appropriate specialists in PGH.

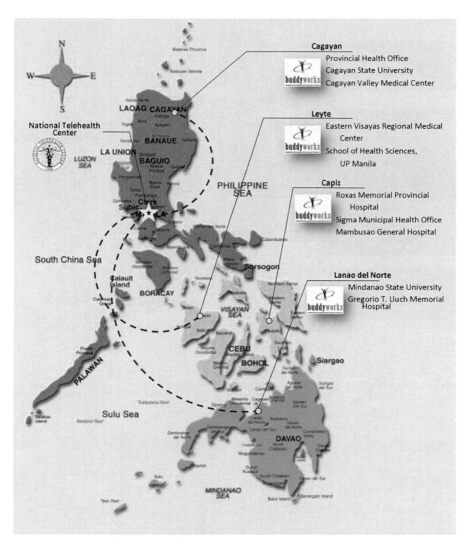

Fig. 8.2 Location of health facilities throughout the country participating in BuddyWorks

8.2.2
Educational Opportunities

Telenursing per se is not yet available in the undergraduate curricula of Philippine nursing schools. However, the Commission on Higher Education (CHED) has already mandated, in its Memorandum Order No. 5s2008 dated 14 March 2008, the inclusion of 36 lecture hours (two units) and 54 laboratory hours (one unit) of nursing informatics for bachelor of science in nursing programs of the more than 400 CHED-recognized nursing schools in the country. The CHED is the Philippine government agency that regulates tertiary-level educational institutions, including nursing schools.

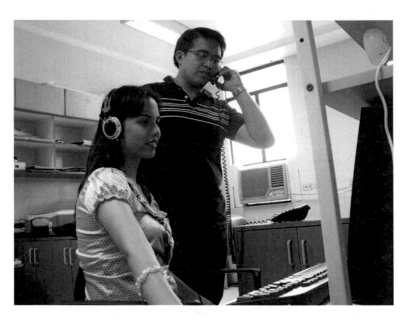

Fig. 8.3 A telenurse operates the BuddyWorks portal as a physician confers remotely with another health professional through the Internet using VoIP

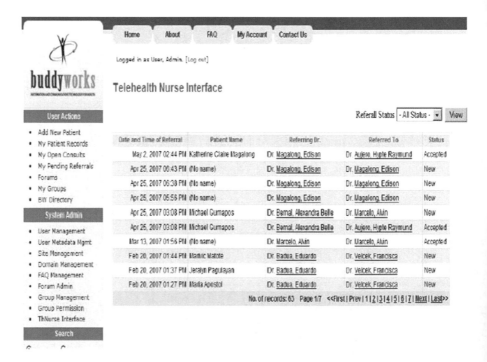

Fig. 8.4 The BuddyWorks portal's telehealth nurse interface

This nursing informatics course deals with the use of information technology (IT) system and data standards based on nursing informatics principles and theories. It further deals with the utilization of clinical information systems in the management and decision making of patient care. Table 8.1 outlines the course.

Table 8.1 Outline of government-mandated nursing informatics course for curricula of Philippine nursing schools

A. Computers and nursing
  1. Computers and nursing
  2. Historical perspectives of nursing and the computer
  3. Electronic health record from a historical perspective

B. Computer system
  1. Computer hardware
  2. Computer software and systems
  3. Open source and free software
  4. Data processing
  5. The Internet: a nursing resource
  6. PDA and wireless devices
  7. Incorporating evidence: use of computer-based clinical decision support system for health professionals

C. Issues in informatics
  1. Nursing informatics and health-care policy
  2. The role of technology in the medication-use process
  3. Health-care data standards
  4. Electronic health record systems: US federal initiatives and public/private partnerships
  5. Dependable systems for quality care
  6. Nursing minimum data set systems

D. Informatics theory
  1. Theories, models, and frameworks
  2. Advanced terminology systems
  3. Implementing and upgrading clinical information systems

E. Practice application
  1. Practice application
  2. Critical care applications
  3. Community health applications
  4. Ambulatory care systems
  5. Internet tools for advanced nursing practice
  6. Informatics solutions for emergency preparedness and response
  7. Vendor applications

F. Administrative application
  1. Administrative applications of IT for nursing managers
  2. Translation of evidence, clinical practice guidelines, and automated implementation tools
  3. Data mining and knowledge discovery

G. Consumer's use of informatics
  1. Consumer and patient use of computers for health
  2. Decision support for consumers

(continued)

Table 8.1 (continued)

H. Educational applications
   1. The nursing curriculum in the information age
   2. Accessible, effective distance education anytime, anywhere
   3. Innovations in telehealth

I. Research application
   1. Computer use in nursing research
   2. Computerized information resources

J. International perspectives
   1. Canada
   2. Europe
   3. Pacific Rim
   4. Asia
   5. South America

K. The future of informatics
   1. Future directions

PDA personal digital assistant

The foregoing is a recent development in nursing education in the country. Previously, nursing students were only taught how to use computers, without training on how this and IT in general relate to nursing practice. This change in the approach to this important aspect of nursing education is the outcome of an international curricular benchmarking conducted by the CHED to ensure that the scope of Philippine nursing education is global and at par with those in other countries. This is in view of the extensive migration of Filipino nurses. Evidently, the Philippine government wants to guarantee that the skilled labor the country is exporting is of high quality.

Paradoxically, while this guarantee may make Filipino nursing graduates in greater demand abroad, it also allows those who do remain to acquire competencies that may overcome any resulting shortage in health manpower resource by way of telenursing, that is to say if we are to regard this and telehealth in general as alternative strategies for addressing the issue of inequitable access to health care. Of course, save for some discussion of innovations in telehealth, the nursing informatics course outlined above does not unequivocally pertain to telenursing, nursing informatics, strictly speaking, being a distinct, although related, field. But clearly, the competencies and know-how it promises to deliver has applications in telenursing.

8.3
Future Directions

The scrapped National Broadband Network project, which aimed to electronically connect all local as well as national government agencies and offices in the country in a high-speed, broadband network,[8] would have gone a long way in facilitating projects like

BuddyWorks that specifically deliver health-care services through the Internet. But all is not lost. Although the status of a legislative bill that would advocate for the use of ICT in delivering health-care services, called the National Telehealth Service Act of 2009, is not clear as of this writing, most recently, the Congressional Commission on Science, Technology and Engineering is looking favorably at the National Telehealth Project being developed by the UP to enable health professionals to remotely manage patients in distant communities.[10]

The UP has developed another computerized information system, an electronic health record system called community health information tracking system (CHITS). CHITS integrates data storage and retrieval for various national health programs. It is already being regularly used by its target beneficiaries, to a much greater extent, in fact, than BuddyWorks, its "sister" telehealth project.

CHITS allows the health personnel within one health center to pass patient and other information back and forth among themselves (see Fig. 8.5). But while in its present form it is still an intra-facility set-up in health centers, it is being studied as a tool for monitoring utilization of out-patient benefits covered by the National Health Insurance Program (NHIP). In line with this, inter-facility connectivity, even on a national scale, is envisioned for the system as this will be necessary if it were to be useful to the NHIP. This would be a scenario for telehealth.

We are already seeing in the Philippines the foundations for increased practice of telenursing. The technology is already available and the necessary manpower already deliverable. Granting that legislative and fiscal prerequisites are met, the stage would be set for this emerging field.

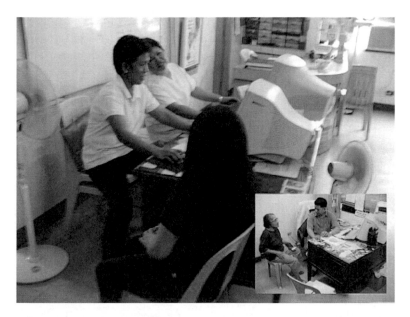

Fig. 8.5 Nurses in a health center entering the result of their initial interview of a patient into CHITS, for subsequent viewing by the center physician (*shown in inset*) through his own computer terminal in his office when he examines the patient

8.4
Summary

- Telenursing is not yet a mainstream profession in the Philippines. However, the archipelagic nature of the country's geography, coupled with a depleting health manpower resource, have compelled health-care providers to use ICT as a means for delivering health, including nursing, services.
- Telehealth is seen as a potential supplementary means of delivering health services to remote communities where doctors, nurses, or other health professionals are either unavailable or lacking.
- UP's telemedicine project, BuddyWorks, involves a web portal through which physicians and other health professionals all over the country collaborate with specialists in the PGH, thus improving health-care services with the use of ICT.
- CHED has mandated the inclusion of 36 lecture hours and 54 laboratory hours of nursing informatics for bachelor of science in nursing programs of CHED-recognized nursing schools in the country. This nursing informatics course deals with the use of information technology (IT) system and data standards based on nursing informatics principles and theories.
- The UP has also developed another computerized information system, CHITS, which integrates data storage and retrieval for various national health programs.

Acknowledgments Special thanks go to Prof. Teresita I. Barcelo, Ph.D., President of the Philippine Nursing Association and Head of the Research and Creative Writing Program of the University of the Philippines College of Nursing, for sharing some insight. Information provided by the CHED, through Ms. Sheila F. Jalbuena of the Office of Programs and Standards, is also much appreciated.

Glossary

Devolution – Transfer of responsibility for the provision of basic services and facilities from the national to the local governments.

District health system – A more or less contained segment of the national health system that comprises a well-defined administrative and geographic area, rural or urban, including all institutions and sectors contained in it whose activities contribute to improve health.

Health center – A primary-care facility in the district health system. It is the government's lowest level of health care in the multi-tiered health referral system.

Information and communication technology – Any technology, including but not limited to IT, for transmitting, communicating, or broadcasting information.

Information technology – Electronic storage, processing, and retrieval of information utilizing computer systems.

Inter-local health zone (area health zone) – Nationally endorsed unit for local health service management and delivery in the Philippines.

Store-and-forward (asynchronous) – A process in telecommunications whereby information is sent to an intermediate station and stored there for subsequent transmission to its final destination or another intermediate station at a later time.

Telehealth/telemedicine – Delivery of health-care services across a distance utilizing ICT. Distinction is sometimes made between telemedicine and telehealth, with the former referring specifically to curative health care and the latter to promotive and preventive care. Telehealth may also be taken or as the umbrella term encompassing all of promotive and preventive as well as curative care. In this chapter, the two terms are used synonymously.

Telenursing – Subset of telehealth/telemedicine pertaining to nursing care.

Triaging – System of sorting patients according to clinical needs.

References

1. Buban CE. WHO calls on states to help avert crisis on health workers. *Philippine Daily Inquirer*. April 8, 2006:B4.
2. Crisostomo S. Health workers warn health care system may collapse. *The Philippine Star*. September 17, 2005:6.
3. Department of Health. *A Handbook on Inter-Local Health Zones: District Health System in a Devolved Setting*. Manila: Department of Health; 2002.
4. Esguerra CV. 56th World Health Day: execs focus on exodus of nurses, docs. *Philippine Daily Inquirer*. April 8, 2006:A16.
5. Lorenzo FME, Dela Rosa JF, Paraso GR, et al. *Migration of Health Workers: Country Case Study Philippines*. Geneva: International Labor Organization; 2006.
6. Maheu MM, Whitten P, Allen A. *E-health, Telehealth, and Telemedicine: A Guide to Start-Up and Success*. San Francisco: Jossey-Bass, Inc.; 2001.
7. Maramba IDC, Marcelo AB. The BuddyWorks telehealth project: best practices and lessons learned. In: Rosario-Braid F, Tuazon RR, Gamolo NO, eds. *A Reader on Information and Communication Technology Planning for Development*. 2nd ed. Manila: Asian Institute of Journalism and Communication; 2007.
8. Ubac ML. GMA: NBN deal is dead. *Philippine Daily Inquirer*. October 3, 2007: Vol. 22, No. 297, p. A1.
9. Valmero A. National telehealth bill mulled. INQUIRER.net, http://newsinfo.inquirer.net/breakingnews/infotech/view/20090225-191026/National-telehealth-bill-mulled. Accessed February 25, 2010.

New Trends in Diagnosis Support and Role of Nurses Based on RIGHT-like Systems

9

Antoni Zwiefka and Kazimierz Frączkowski

Abbreviations

eHR	Electronic Health Record
EU	European Union
GP	General Practitioner
ICT	Information and Communication Technology
IT	Information Technology

9.1
Background/Nursing Practice in Europe

The creation of the informational society has an influence on expectation and form of the role of nurses; moreover, there is an influence on the concept of nurses itself. However, the major principles and concepts of it do not change during the last decade. Apart from it, the main purpose of nurses is to take care of people, granting the help, and preventing illnesses. The changes that took place in the society have an influence on caretaking of all ill people. Not only working conditions, but also the roles of nurses were changed. The foundation of inspiration and new trends that took place in an informational society are features, functions, and jurisdictions of an informational society. These changes favor the improvement of a medical treatment. The role of nurses is the main element because of the fact that the society is becoming older. In 1994, the information society was created in Europe. At this time the report that was written by Bangemann (Europe and the Global Information Society) was published. This report became the proximate cause of public discussion about information society. Ten initiatives were proposed in order to develop new techniques in the following areas:

A. Zwiefka (✉)
The Marshal's Office of Lower Silesia, Wybrzeże J. Słowackiego 12-14, 50-411 Wroclaw, Poland
e-mail: azwiefka@umwd.pl

S. Kumar and H. Snooks (eds.), *Telenursing*, Health Informatics,
DOI: 10.1007/978-0-85729-529-3_9, © Springer-Verlag London Limited 2011

- Telework
- Outside training
- Network linking universities and laboratories
- Tele-information service for small and medium enterprises
- Management of road traffic
- Control of airline traffic
- Computerization of public order
- Trans-European network of public administration
- Information highway for metropolitan areas

Two years later, the so-called green book titled *Living and Working in Information Society* was published. It shows the consequences of transformation, which have great influence on life in a society.

"New aim of building information society" was introduced in all of the e-Europe projects. It exploits new economy. In 1999, the green book titled *Public Sector Information: A Key Resource for Europe* was published. It provides benefits for society by using telecommunication and informative technologies. The plan of building a new society was passed in Liverpool (23–24 March 2000) in "The Lisbon Strategy." In 2000, during the meeting in Feira the plan of e-Europe was accepted. In Gothenburg, the plan, which conceded the modernization and accelerated the reform in countries that wanted to become the members of European Union was accepted. During the summit in Seville (spain), the plan of e-Europe was accepted. This plan obliges countries to:

- Develop an electronic system
- Introduce an electronic health service
- Assure the access to the Internet

In the summit of European Faculty during May 2005 the program of "European Information Society 2010" was accepted. Because of this program, information technology causes the development of the information society. Europe strives for creation of global information society. The main characteristics of information society are the following:

- Creation of information – global generation, requirement, and use of information
- Downloading of information – the possibility of downloading information by everyone
- Striation of information – development of technologies for gathering information
- Conversion of information – handing over information regardless of time and place
- Using information – unlimited usage of information and the Internet

Information society has to meet the following functions:

- Education – popularization of the scientific knowledge and education
- Communication – information society should provide communication among different global groups

- Socialization and activation – mobilization of temporarily or permanently disabled people in the society; enhancing possibility of working at home and activating disabled people
- Participation – possibility of discussion and voting on the Internet
- Organization contention market
- Security and control – security of citizens and institutions against virtual crime

9.2
Current Telenursing Practice

Telenursing is a usage of telecommunication and information technologies in health-care field when there is a large distance between a nurse and a patient. Telenursing is a part of the European Union program called telehealth. This program focuses on the help, which can be obtained by telecommunication technology or more complicated technologies, e.g., video-conferences. Telenursing is connected with the role of nurses in using new techniques in dealing with a patient. Specific form of telenursing is connected with the usage of electro-magnetic canals, e.g., radio or optic, to send voice, data, signals, and videocommunications.

At community homes, telenursing relies on usage systems that enable one to monitor physiological parameters such as blood pressure, level of glucose, measure, and weight. By the interactive video systems, patients can contact a nurse at any time and organize videoconsultations in order to clarify problems such as changing of dressing or rediscuss the level of insulin. It enables nurses to obtain correct and updated information. The continuity of health care will be provided by contacting patients. New technologies give nurses the access to education[5,9,10] through videoconferences, multimedia lectures, and distance learning. It is possible to train clinical skills and practice them by simulation of patient behavior.

- There will be less need for hospital beds because of more consideration taken over by general practitioner (GP) and teleconsulting centers.[11]
- Children who live with aged people will be included in telenursing.
- There will be more need for palliative treatment because of the large number of aged people who need health care.[4]

9.2.1
Evolution of the EU Opinion on Nursing

Currently, telenursing is in the initial stage of development as separate scientific field within telehealth. As in other disciplines, the professionals accomplish their actions. They fulfill a great mission within the health care. The development of education and practice, as well as nurses' investigation is highly necessary to develop this discipline. All matters that are connected with nurses' practice are taken into consideration.

There are elaborated models that can answer the questions: what are nursing? What exactly a nurse is? What is a nurse's occupation? The creation of nursing models is connected with scientific attitude to this field of knowledge. One of them is understanding nursing as an art, which requires qualifications and ability to do it. It is the occupation that requires mental skills, working order and knowledge, and professional experience. New informational technological communication is developing and it is the foundation of telemedicine and telecare, what is more it is connected with telenursing as a model of execution of this occupation. This model is connected with old method of treatment, where patients were treated at their homes (Fig. 9.1).

European Union is changing its point of view about health care among aged people. In the agency's register (26 February 2008) is included the opinion of regional committee: "the comfortable function of older people in the informational society." It can be read as follows:

- The regional committee claims that ICT project, which proposes self-reliant life and remote control of health should improve services and ensure more time for work. Technology should be accommodated to older people. It cannot lead to loneliness and it has to respect the privacy and dignity of older people.
- The committee supports the plan to 2007 and 2008 accomplish the political review. The main aim will be supporting skills which are necessary to use digital technology. Supporting local and regional government in overusing structural fangs should be the priority. "Learning for all life" should be supported as well in order to develop older people's skills and using valuable experiences from other people (mainly mobile phones and the Internet), which changed language, culture, media, and society as a whole.[5] However, the problem of informational "gap" concerns wider range of issues than possibility of using computer. One of the solutions could be projects which engage young and old together.

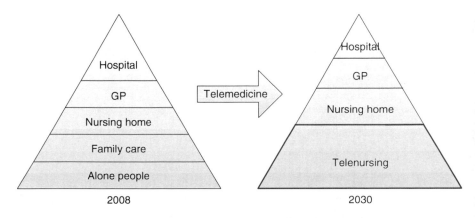

Fig. 9.1 Change of the health-care model by increasing the role of telenursing

9.3
Future Direction

"4 leaf clover" is a project under the Lifelong Learning Programme, which is supported by EU Leonardo da Vinci. Addressee of this project is staff connected with senior services. There are many opportunities in pursuing lifelong learning in this sector. Partners involved in those activities are from Denmark, Portugal, Poland, Germany, Italy, and the UK.[1,8]

The project shows directions in which the sector of senior services will develop in Europe in future. The ICT and mechanical/electronic devices, besides providing elderly with enhanced mobility, improved senses and practical help, can also change the work of the caregivers. The report of assistive technologies and lifelong learning shows the newest groundbreaking technologies. The crucial point is that advanced technologies provide both challenges and new opportunities for caregivers' lifelong learning. ICT is becoming more and more universal, flexible, and interactive. To make the best use of technology, the senior service staff need to increase their competencies. As technologies are changing and developing continuously, there is a need to give lifelong learning opportunities a higher priority. Lifelong learning not only is connected with providing a formal course, but also helps to shift attention away from traditional teaching activities to acquire new skills and knowledge through more comprehensive learning process.

Computers and IT are dominating the eldercare sector as well as other health-care sectors, especially in administrative field. It helps to plan time consumption in a proper way and optimize the services delivered in home care and nursing homes; to increase the efficiency, work planning has become more rigid. The implementation of administrative technologies in the care sector seems to follow the same phases as seen in other sectors: first a rationalization phase, then a flexibilization phase, and finally a service enhancement phase. In this phase, existing work processes are computerized, for example, booking, planning, and documentation. Information about medical issues can also be computerized so as to create a better overview and safer medication procedures. Flexibilization phase of the systems will be opened up for a wider communication between the eldercare management and the caregivers. The caregivers can be given tools to undertake the detailed work planning themselves. They can also use the system to collect information that they need in specific situations, for example, information about medication and follow-up on hospital treatments. The caregivers can add information of importance for other caregivers. The division of work between skilled nurses and caregivers might gradually be altered. Information access can lead to higher proficiency among personnel with lower qualifications and bring a higher level of safety in the operations when information is codified accessible in new ways. New services phase of technology is further developed to an extent where the users might also experience a better quality of service. There is a platform included for the user's interaction – the elderly will be able to communicate with the care system and caregivers. As a consequence, the character of the service will change entirely and the users will be better informed and empowered. A good example is that with the help of this system the elderly patients/clients will be informed when the caregivers are expected to come and check the patients' medical records. Everybody can observe health symptoms, but to verify health problems or to monitor risk factors most people need help from medical experts. However, very rapidly the self-diagnosis and self-monitoring systems are emerging. They can help patients to be prepared for consultations with doctors or to provide a basis for a second opinion. A continuous or frequent health-monitoring system may shorten the time between suspicion of illness and treatment, which is generally life and cost saving. Self-diagnoses and health monitoring may also have a function as a preventive measure. Recently, it has been possible to purchase genetic tests, which conclude about dispositions for various deceases, such as Parkinson's, breast and prostate cancer, heart attacks, etc. The tests are hardly definitive, but they may help people with dispositions to undertake necessary lifestyle changes.

9.3.1
New Technologies as a Support in Diagnosis on an Example of RIGHT System

New technologies are fundamental for health informatics or medical informatics, which is the intersection of information science, computer science, and health care. Information skills are necessary for good medical practice. The dynamics of communicating with patients and colleagues are altered when the exchange moves from a face-to-face interaction. The patient will stay at home and he or she will communicate through the Internet or telephone. Demographic changes are an essential factor in the implementation of such projects like the program RIGHT. The RIGHT-like system aims at integrating all information needed for the health services. Furthermore, this system will become the platform, which will enable consultation and experts' discussion in each given medical field. Advances in new technologies related to telediagnostics will support medical services. These services will consist in monitoring of life parameters and providing long-distance therapy and rehabilitation. Information skills are basic to good medical practice. Every clinician needs to understand the principles of data interpretation, the logical foundations of the diagnostic process, and the management of uncertainty in clinical knowledge. The problem-oriented medical record is just an information instrument, and clinicians need to know when it is appropriate and when indeed other formulations might be better choices. The dynamics of communicating with patients and colleagues are altered when the exchange moves from a face-to-face interaction to the telephone, e-mail, voicemail, or video. In result of the development of telecommunication, medicine gains a new approach to population and civilization diseases. Then, there was created Telemedicine-Telecare, which prevents the deterioration of living conditions of elderly people. That will improve their mental comfort connected with staying and functioning at home. Therefore, in order to provide proper actions, such solutions should be introduced, among others, which will consider changes connected with aging of the society.

Demographic changes are an essential factor in the implementation of such projects like RIGHT. Each year, there is a decrease in the number of children born; however, the average life expectancy grows. According to demographers, the process of aging of the society, which began in 2005, will reach its maximum between the years 2010 and 2020. In the next decade, around two million people altogether will attain retirement age (women – 60, men – 65). These persons were born during the post-war years (1950s). In 2004, persons aged 65 and older constituted 13.1% of the population (13.3% in Lower Silesia). According to demographers in 2020, 8,200,000 persons will be entitled to pension services (in Poland in 2000 there were 5,700,000 pensioners). It is expected that in 2030, persons aged 65 and older will constitute 23.8% of the population. For each 100 persons in the productive age there will be 70 persons in the unproductive age – children, youth, and older persons.[6]

9.3.2
Can System RIGHT Help Elderly People?

RIGHT, as the real-time intelligent electronic system, has to make up the support for the health-care experts in the range of the quality and pertinence of medical diagnosis and treatment for new member states of the EU. Its aim is to be reached, for Lower Silesia, through the implementation of the computer system, which helps doctors with electronic documentation, in the process of diagnosing and treatment. Medical data gathered in the electronic health record (eHR) will be stored in the central or local medical database using special software based on the newest achievements from the range of semantics and artificial intelligence for the analysis of described cases. Results of such analysis, based on eHR, will be automatically made available for doctors. In this range, the RIGHT project is based on the cooperation with the e-Health program, one of the main programs in the EU, which aims at improving the quality of access to health services also for people residing outside the academic centers.

The RIGHT system aims at integrating all information needed for the health services. Furthermore, this system will become the platform which will enable consultation and experts' discussion in each given medical field. This means that it is designed to perform two main functions: semantic, for finding the information, and helping in accuracy of making diagnostic decisions. In this way, the RIGHT project will support the knowledge of health service professionals and contribute to the enlargement of efficiency and effectiveness, and it will also indirectly influence the efficiency of the whole structure of the health-care system. RIGHT will also contribute to the development of one of the most important questions,[12] namely the European Health Care System. As this system has a modular structure, it suggests that it may be developed for new modules to support the needs of elderly people, including telemedicine modules.

9.3.3
Communication Skills Supporting Elderly People

Therefore, the need for medical services will increase owing to wider use of the ICT technology. These services will consist in monitoring of life parameters and leading long-distance therapy and rehabilitation. The patient will stay at home and he or she will communicate through the Internet or telephone with the teleconsulting center or the GP, who will be able to provide medical services of the highest standard through the use of the RIGHT system. Evolution from current telecommunication technologies to future services of "intelligent environment" should be based on the possible good practices. This brings together a number of examples that have been chosen with the objective of providing some services. New technologies should help disabled and elderly people with new remote services by user participation in technology. The main aim is to give services according to the current trends. Possible impact on people with physical, sensory, or cognitive restrictions may be due to a disability, aging, or the special conditions or equipment they use. New technologies can help elderly people and people with disabilities.[2] To support human navigation and the possibilities for the near future, it possible to develop devices to help people with physical, sensorial, or cognitive restrictions. Techniques for sensoring, positioning, mapping, and navigating can navigate outdoors and indoors. New communication technologies are already available. Elderly people and people with disabilities can be supported by sustained advanced services. In RIGHT system, this new relay services, virtual communities, and enhanced communication are successfully applied.

9.3.4
Telemedicine Aspects

Telecare came into being for the improvement of mentally disabled people's life, allowing them to break through to the recovery of abilities and human potential. Starting from 1965, there has been created the environment, which, through the organization of the center, causes that the employee and customers together can achieve their objectives. Telecare[2] is based on the set of sensors or monitors and controls, which in case of exceeding the specified range, inform about it through the alarm connected to the warning system (or alarm system) of the control center. The large number of the configuration of equipment and answers is possible. Telecare in England consists of a wide range of uses in the range of equipment and services, which alarm the systems controlling life parameters (e.g., checking the blood pressure).[7,9] The immediate help can be obtained either by a direct visit or another form of contact with a doctor. The increase of services accessibility was possible through the development of radio technology and telephony. The measurement of blood pressure and different life parameters can be made using small electronic devices and transferring the results to the telecommunication control center. There are various generations of these technologies at present (Fig. 9.2):

- First generation – the device handy or different alarms
- Second generation – monitoring the house
- Third generation – the mobile and wireless technology

The work includes identifying environment of IT projects execution, pointing out the causes of software projects' failures, and showing the overall impact of the project team on the IT undertakings. Hospitals and health sector institutions will have to undergo transformation process. Regional program called e-health has to propagate and provide IT services using integrated information and communication system supporting both administration and medical services and telediagnostics.[3,4]

Due to the expectations of the best possible health care and the increasing role of nurses in it, the demands concerning nurses' knowledge have been growing rapidly. Nurses are the biggest group among employees in health service who have higher education. Changes that take place in health care have an influence on dynamic rise of role of nurses. Nursing is a powerful force in a health-care system. There are changes in nursing. These are caused by awareness of performing their duties. The occupational autonomy means the best and the

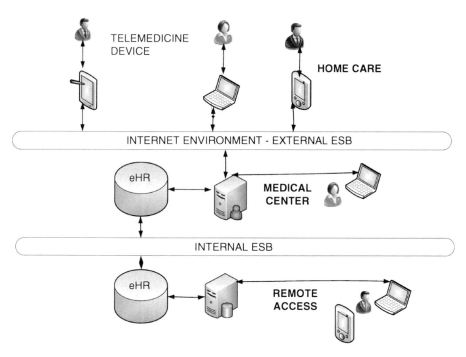

Fig. 9.2 The technical model of telecommunication in telenursing

most professional execution of an occupation within the therapeutic group. It also means working in a group, making self-reliant decisions and nursing. Nurses are not only expected to activate elderly people. The occupational autonomy involves taking responsibility and nurses are fully aware of it. The twenty-first century is a new challenge for nurses, which they can fulfill because they have awareness and they are professionally educated; what is more they have specific knowledge of the subject and required experience.

With the attraction of a growing market more and more companies will be marketing devices in the near future that can be accessed by elderly people and people with disabilities. These concepts in RIGHT-like systems are interpreted in diverse ways. Speaking is the main way of communication between people.[12] Nevertheless, a number of users with disabilities experience restrictions in their speech ability that limit their natural oral communication skills. So, the communication module can support communication between doctors and patients, although it was created for communication between doctors only. In future, telecommunication services can be used for providing remote support that is tuned to the needs of specific groups of people with disabilities. For instance, in RIGHT, it includes reading texts aloud for people with sight restrictions, and controlling devices. According to the demographic aspect RIGHT-like systems can be very important in health-care system. Now, there is 14–23 GPs per 10,000 patients and one doctor can spend 5–10 min per patient. Demographic prognoses suggest that in future it will be much worse. That is why the RIGHT-like system can help doctors make Polish health-care system more efficient. It is also possible to make some more modules in future and it will support telemedicine, so patient can stay at home and be diagnosed.[9]

9.3.5
Mechanical and Electronic Devices for Health Monitoring

Some of the devices are used to monitor diseases that are already diagnosed and where the patient is under treatment. The purpose of a personal device in the home or on the body is to allow the patient to adjust the treatment themselves, or to see a doctor if the monitoring shows alarming signals. A number of devices have been available for several years and new and improved tools are entering the market regularly. New instruments in telemedicine are increasing the possibilities dramatically. Welfare gains can be obtained in the sense that the elderly people can stay at home instead of being hospitalized and still receive medical supervision. Incidences can be discussed with doctors faster than if the patients have to be transported to the hospital. Robots have potential for the entertainment and companionship of the elderly. Japanese citizens are more apt at personalizing the technical instruments than Westerners usually are. A Japanese nursing home has implemented "roboteddies" with a variety of functions. Some even have integrated sensors with a role in terms of monitoring the well-being of the elderly. A personal robot not only is able to assist the elderly by collecting information, doing housework, etc., but it can also mobilize the user in a way that fits the physical conditions and needs for exercise and training. Robots are likely to be used further in rehabilitation, as "personal" trainers for those who are regaining strength after, for example, a fracture of a limb. Such robots have already entered hospitals, but there is a need to personalize and adapt them for use in private homes and nursing homes.

Over some decades it has been an established element in social policies that the elderly should remain in their own houses for as long as possible.[1] Different types of supervision and communication instruments help to postpone the time where it is necessary for an elderly person to move to a nursing home. Supervision is also an element in terms of letting people out of hospitals faster, or in avoiding hospitalization altogether. Sensors are being developed and improved rapidly, and they are applied in many situations. They can register temperature, pressure, airborne substances, light, etc. Sensors may be placed on the body, in clothes, or anywhere in the environment of the elderly. A sensor for intelligent bandages has been introduced. It measures humidity, temperature, and bacteria. The bandage is in electronic connection with the health center. A faster and more targeted healing may take place and the patient can stay at home. In principle, the patient may even follow the healing process on his/her own computer.

9.4
Summary

- The plan of building a new society was passed in Liverpool (23–24 March 2000) in "The Lisbon Strategy." In the summit of European Faculty during May 2005 the program of "European Information Society 2010" was accepted.
- Telenursing is a part of the European Union program called telehealth. This program focuses on helping patients contact nurses when required through telecommunication technology or more complicated technologies, e.g., videoconferences.

- European Union is changing its point of view about health care among aged people. In the agency's register (26 February 2008) is included the opinion of regional committee: "the comfortable function of older people in the informational society."
- The RIGHT system aims to integrate all information needed for the health services. The RIGHT project will support the knowledge of health service professionals and contribute to the enlargement of efficiency and effectiveness, and it will also indirectly influence the efficiency of the whole structure of the health-care system.
- RIGHT also contributes to the development of sustained advanced services for supporting the needs of elderly people and people with disabilities.

Acknowledgments   We would like to express our gratitude to all those who supported us in our research work. We would like to thank them for all their help, support, interest, and valuable hints. We are especially obliged to Professor Bernard Richards.

Glossary

Electronic health record (eHR) – eHR it is a record in digital format that is capable of being shared across different health care settings, by being embedded in network-connected enterprise-wide information systems.

General practitioner (GP) – GP is a medical practitioner who treats acute and chronic illness and provides preventive care and health education for all ages and both sexes.

Information computing technology (ICT) – ICT consists of all technical means used to handle information and aid communication, including both computer and network hardware, as well as necessary software.

Intelligent environments – Intelligent environments are spaces with embedded systems and information and communication technologies creating interactive spaces that bring computation into the physical world.

Telecare – Telecare is a term given to offering remote care of old and physically less-able people, providing the care and reassurance needed to allow them to remain living in their own homes.

Telehealth – Telehealth is the delivery of health-related services and information via telecommunications technologies.

Tele-information – Tele-information services are based on an alliance of digital telecommunication and computer technology that play an important role in interhuman communications.

Telemedicine – Telemedicine is a rapidly developing application of clinical medicine where medical information is transferred through interactive audiovisual media for the purpose of consulting, and sometimes remote medical procedures or examinations.

Telenursing – Telenursing refers to the use of telecommunications and information technology for providing nursing services in health care whenever a large physical distance exists between patient and nurse, or between any number of nurses.

Telework – Telework is a work arrangement in which employees enjoy flexibility in working location and hours.

References

1. Joint Publication. An Ageing Europe. Assistive technologies and lifelong learning report. Leonardo da Vinci Project no. 134320-LLP-2007-DK-LMP; 2009.
2. Curry RG, Trejo Tinoco M, Wardle D. Telecare: using information and communication technology to support independent living by older, disabled and vulnerable people; UK Health Department Report; 2003. Available from http://www.telecare.org.uk/shared_asp_files/GFSR. asp?NodeID=46395 accessed May 7th, 2011.
3. Frączkowski K. Model of mapping activities and competence ICT project. *Ann Inf.* 2006;4: 86-103.
4. Frączkowski K. Model informatyzacji placówek ochrony zdrowia oraz wyzwania dotyczące e-Zdrowia. *Acta BioOptima Informatica Med Inżynieria Biomedyczna.* 2006;12:120-124.
5. Hastie T, TibshiramiT FJ. *The Elements of Statistical Learning. Springer Series in Statistics.* Heidelberg: Springer; 2001.
6. Hyde RB. Facilitative communication skills training: social support for elderly people. *Gerontologist.* 1988;28(3):418-420.
7. Jonsson AM, Willman A. Implementation of telenursing within home healthcare. *Telemed J E Health.* 2008;14(10):1057-1062.
8. Joint Publication. An Ageing Europe. Professional profiles in European senior service sector typology and expected changes report. Leonardo da Vinci Project no. 134320-LLP-2007-DK-LMP; 2009.
9. Satava R, Angood PB, et al. The physiologic cipher at altitude. Telemedicine and real-time monitoring of climbers on Mount Everest. *Telemed J Health.* 2000;6(3):303-313.
10. Snooks HA, Williams AM, et al. Red nursing? The development of telenursing aim. *J Adv Nurs.* 2008;61(6):631-640.
11. Wyke A. *Medycyna przyszłości. Telemedycyna, Cyberchirurgia i nasze szanse na nieśmiertelność.* Warszawa: Pruszyński i S-ka; 2003.
12. Zwiefka A, Klakocar J, Maroszek J, et al. Zastosowanie nowych technologii w ochronie zdrowia w celu redukcji ryzyka diagnozy i leczenia. *Przewodnik lekarza.* 2008;1(103): 281-286.

Telenursing in Chronic Respiratory Diseases

10

Carlos Zamarrón, Emilio Morete, and Francisco Gonzalez

Abbreviations

COPD   Chronic Obstructive Pulmonary Disease
FTP   File Transfer Protocol
HRQoL   Health-related Quality of Life
IT   Information Technology
PCC   Primary Care Centers
PDA   Personal Digital Assistant
SAS   Sleep Apnea Syndrome
SBK   Systems Based on Knowledge
SF36   Medical Outcomes Study Short Form-36
SGRQ   Saint George Respiratory Questionnaire

10.1
Background

Patients with long-term conditions such as chronic pulmonary diseases represent a major health-care problem for the public health-care systems. Among these conditions are the sleep apnea syndrome (SAS), neuromuscular diseases with respiratory involvement, and chronic obstructive pulmonary disease (COPD). A recent study showed that over 27,000 people died from COPD in 2004 in the UK, and that caring for these patients represented a cost of 6.6 billion pounds for the UK national health-care system.[7,8] The spiraling health-care budgets and the economic downturn we are facing in our days are forcing health-care providers to look for new cost-effective solutions to

C. Zamarrón (✉)
Service of Neumology, Complejo Hospitalario Universitario de Santiago de Compostela,
c/Travesia Choupana s/n, E-15706 Santiago de Compostela, Spain
e-mail: carlos.zamarron.sanz@sergas.es

S. Kumar and H. Snooks (eds.), *Telenursing*, Health Informatics,
DOI: 10.1007/978-0-85729-529-3_10, © Springer-Verlag London Limited 2011

provide the best possible care. Information technology (IT) and particularly the new ways of delivering care remotely through telecare interventions seem to be a pivotal aspect in this question.[19] IT can be implemented as web-based applications,[9,10] mobile phone and alert systems,[17,23] or telephone and videoconferencing to be used with chronic patients who are at their homes.[5,13]

Patients with chronic respiratory diseases frequently have exacerbations of their condition. While some impairments remain unreported[16] others end up in visits to the emergency department, which eventually very often result in hospitalization.[1] It has been reported that about one-third of these patients will be seen again or admitted to hospital within the subsequent 2 months.[25] A good home control of patients with chronic respiratory diseases will make possible early detection of exacerbations of their condition, which in turn would reduce hospital admissions and slow disease progression.[27]

There are a number of personnel involved in a telehomecare setting suitable for use in patients with chronic pulmonary diseases. Among them physicians and nurses are probably the most relevant. Most studies regarding the use of telemedicine are assessed from a physician or a technological point of view. However, despite nursing staff playing a relevant role in providing health-care services to these patients, they are commonly neglected in these studies. The use of IT for providing nursing services in health care is commonly known as telenursing. As a field, it is part of telehealth, which is in many aspects related to other telemedical procedures, such as telediagnosis, teleconsultation, or telemonitoring.

Telenursing is growing rapidly in many countries, due to factors such as concerns for reducing the costs of health care and an increase in the number of aging and chronically ill patients, and to increase health-care coverage to remote regions. One of the most distinctive telenursing applications is homecare. For example, patients who are immobilized, live in remote places, and have chronic ailments or disabling diseases may stay at home and be "visited" and assisted regularly by a nurse via videoconferencing, Internet, videophone, etc. Among its many benefits, telenursing may help solve the shortage of nurses, save travel time, and keep patients out of hospital. Here, we describe our experience with three telemedicine settings aimed for patients with chronic respiratory diseases, emphasizing the nursing involvement.

10.2
Telenursing in Respiratory Diseases

10.2.1
Sleep Apnea Syndrome

Telenursing will make it possible to provide care for a greater number of people who suffer from sleep-disordered breathing. Treating these patients is relevant for a number of reasons, among them an increased risk in terms of traffic and work-related accidents or an increased cardiovascular risk. As a result of the high prevalence of SAS, screening strategies must be implemented to identify high-risk populations. Sleep units are currently overcrowded while demand continues growing; therefore, solutions must be found that are more widely applicable than conventional polysomnography. Alternatives are needed to reduce costs and waiting lists.[4] One of these alternatives could be unsupervised home-based polygraphic studies[20] or home oximetry,[28] which could be under control of nursing staff.

In recent years, new telemedicine procedures have been tested to diagnose and treat SAS. For example, remote polysomnography monitoring has been tested as an alternative to conventional polysomnography by Kristo et al.[15] who used a conventional FTP Internet file transfer system to transmit data. The procedure proved to be technically and clinically feasible, cost-effective, and clinically useful for improving patient accessibility to the sleep units.[14,15] Pelletier-Fleury et al.[22] compared a system of home-recorded polysomnography with respect to polysomnography using a telemedicine system in terms of diagnosing the SAS. These authors compared the effectiveness and costs of both systems in 99 consecutive patients and found that the polysomnography telerecordings were ineffective in 11.2%, while home-recorded polysomnography was ineffective in 23.4%. However, telerecordings were more expensive than domiciliary recordings. Therefore, the implementation of a strategy based on a home-recorded polysomnography system appears to be cheaper than the telemonitoring strategy.[6,21,22]

For the last 4 years we carried out a study on 300 patients with SAS in our institution involving three primary care centers (PCCs) and the sleep clinic of our hospital. In our setting, the patient with possible SAS first is seen by the general practitioner at the PCC where a presumed diagnosis is made. Then, patient is asked to take home a pulse oximeter (Criticare Systems Inc., Waukesha, WI, USA), a sleep questionnaire, and an Epworth Sleepiness Scale.[12] The nurse in charge of these procedures shows the patient how to use the device and how to fill the forms. The next day the patient returns the pulse oximeter together with the filled forms and the nurse proceeds to transfer the data from the pulse oximeter to a conventional computer to produce a plain text format file containing all measurements made by the device overnight. This file, together with the scores resulting from the filled forms, is forwarded to the sleep clinic, which is in our hospital (Fig. 10.1). Here, another nurse reads the data and proceeds to discriminate those patients under no risk of suffering from SAS (normal oxygen saturation and Epworth score below 12) from those at risk of having SAS. This is an important step because only those patients who meet the criteria are transferred to the physician. Then, the physician will determine whose patients should be transferred to the hospital to undergo a full study of their condition. For this, the patients are admitted to the hospital for one night and while sleeping a polysomnography study is performed. This includes electroencephalography, electrooculography, electromyography, electrocardiography, oxygen saturation, heart rate, respiratory movements, and oronasal flow.

A constant communication between the nurse at the PCC, and the nurse and the doctor at the sleep clinic helps to solve sporadic problems regarding how to categorize the patients or how to handle the possible problems with the recordings. The role of the nursing staff in this setting is relevant because they are the first stage in the screening of patients with SAS and save hours of more expensive labor time of the physicians. We estimated that these procedures have reduced about 20% of hospital admissions to perform polysomnography studies in our institution. The data are safely protected because we use a private Internet network with proper encryption, which is part of our public health system.

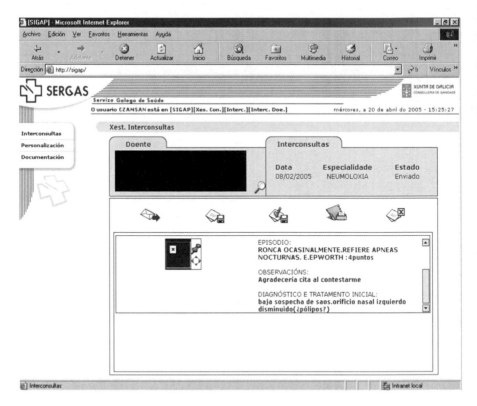

Fig. 10.1 Sample of a screen window of the physician and nurse interface for control of SAS patients. This interface allows downloading the data of a selected patient for further study

10.2.2
Neuromuscular Diseases

Neuromuscular diseases associated with chronic respiratory failure share certain aspects such as weakness of respiratory muscles, progression toward chronic respiratory failure, and the eventual appearance of episodes of acute respiratory failure. Patients with neuromuscular diseases are usually young and willing to use IT. These conditions cause several limitations that may be improved with a telemedicine system, such as functional limitation and dependency associated with muscular weakness, the insidious development of respiratory failure, and the frequent episodes of acute respiratory failure.

In our hospital, we evaluated a telemedicine system for home telemonitoring three patients with neuromuscular diseases that need assisted ventilation with a mechanical ventilator. In these patients, cardiorespiratory variables (oxygen saturation, heart rate, and blood pressure) or electrocardiogram can be recorded at home (Fig. 10.2). Also videoconference between the patient and health-care personnel is possible. For this, we used a Seguitel system platform (Telefonica SA, Madrid) intended for patient homecare and based on conventional computers and servers, and can be accessed by a web interface.

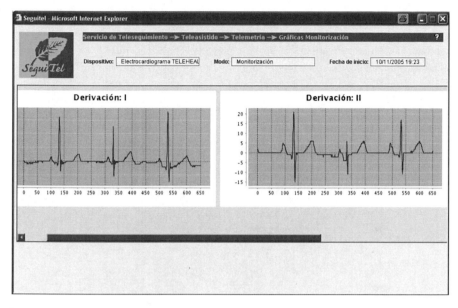

Fig. 10.2 Home telemonitoring system. Electrocardiogram as seen by the nurse or the physician at the reference hospital. All recorded data can be displayed on the screen computer. The figure shows derivations I and II of one of our patients with a neuromuscular disease. The data can be retrieved off-line for subsequent analysis

The main advantage of using a web interface is the ability to connect to the server from any computer or personal digital assistant (PDA) equipped with a web browser. A Firewall avoids unauthorized access. In addition to providing security, the user-password procedure identifies the roll of the person involved. The system is designed to be accessed basically by three different users: the patient, the physician, and the nurse.

The patient may interact with the system at any time. Most interactions are mainly related to input the biomedical data requested by the doctor or the nurse who is in charge of the patient. The patient has access to a simple menu that is displayed on a regular TV-set screen that can be accessed via a small wireless device. There are a number of devices installed at the patient's home for recording vital parameters (pulse oximeter, sphygmomanometer, and electrocardiograph). Instructions on how to obtain and send the clinical data can be requested to the system and they appear on the TV screen. The patients are also equipped with a wireless device (alarm button) that can generate an alarm in the system. The Internet access is used to transmit the data with good quality and at a reasonable cost.

The physician has the responsibility of the patient follow-up and requests the appropriate clinical tests. Periodically by means of videoconference the physician interacts with the patient to keep track of the patient's condition. The physician can also interact with the system through a web interface where test results and clinical data can be visualized, patient alarms (requests for assistance) can be attended, videoconferences are held, and, in general, the patient follow-up is managed.

The nurse visits the patient at home once a month. Once at home, the nurse performs all regular procedures as if the patient was not telemonitored and then checks whether the equipment and communications are working properly. These tests include testing all medical (sphygmomanometer, electrocardiograph, pulse oximeter, and mechanical ventilator) and communication devices. If a malfunction is observed, the problem is reported to the physician who is in charge of the patient. Every 2 weeks the nurse connects via videoconference with the patient, confirms that the system is working correctly and checks the clinical parameters. If the patient's condition worsens, the oxygen saturation is monitored overnight (Fig. 10.3) and reported next morning to the physician by the nurse. If the measurements are abnormal, the physician is informed and instructions to the patient's family

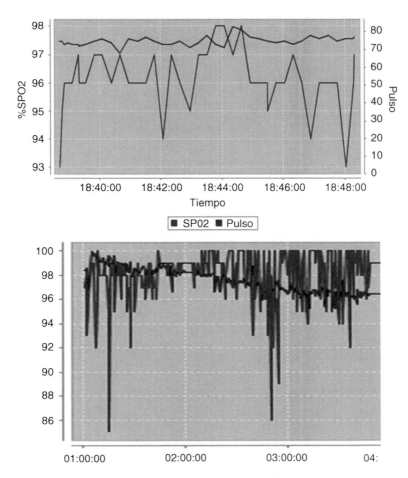

Fig. 10.3 Data recorded using our home telemonitoring system. *Top*: the graph shows the oxygen saturation (*red line*) and the heart rate (*blue line*) recorded during 8 min (from 18:40 to 18:48). *Below*: The same data as above but here the recording time lasted 3 h while the patient was sleeping (from 1:00 to 4:00). Data was obtained from a patient with amyotrophic lateral sclerosis under mechanical ventilation

are given to change the ventilator parameters if needed. These procedures are performed every time the patient requests a consultation, which can be made any time.

10.2.3
Chronic Obstructive Pulmonary Disease

COPD is a progressive and largely irreversible condition resulting in breathlessness, cough, and sputum. As the disease progresses, subjects with COPD experience increasing deterioration of their health-related quality of life (HRQoL), with greater impairment in their ability to work and declining participation in social and physical activities. COPD patients who experience more frequent exacerbations present deteriorated in HRQoL as measured by quality-of-life questionnaires. Usually exacerbations are characterized by an increase in dyspnea along with episodes of increase in frequency of cough, the amount of sputum and ronchi, or changes in sputum color. Important management strategies are smoking cessation, vaccinations, rehabilitation, and drug therapy.

Spirometry is a basic test of pulmonary function. The new spirometers that are portable, easy to use, able to store vast amounts of information, and able to transmit results electronically from the patient's home to a health center had great impact in this technique.[2,11] Spirometry studies for diagnosis and follow-up of patients with respiratory diseases are usually made in the pulmonary function laboratory. Nevertheless, this test can also be carried out as an outpatient procedure and the results can later be sent to the laboratory. A number of studies have demonstrated that there is little difference between the diagnostic value of laboratory and ambulatory spirometry.[5]

Preserving a satisfactory quality of life is considered one of the main objectives of health care. Thus, treatment strategies for chronic diseases should aim at improving quality of life as well as survival. Among these conditions affecting quality of life, COPD seems to merit special attention. Patients with advanced COPD sometimes develop respiratory failure. In COPD, telemedicine has been applied for homecare patients and control domiciliary oxygen and ventilation therapy in cases of stable disease. Outpatient care can help reduce hospital stay because home monitoring of respiratory function can facilitate early discharge and delay hospital admissions. The technology currently available allows this type of health assistance, which is supported by a considerable amount of positive experiences.[3,18,24,26]

In order to see the impact that the nursing home visits to patients with COPD could have, we started, some years ago, a pilot program to control these patients at home. This program combined homecare management and easy access to hospital resources and included scheduled nurse home visits as well as patient care on demand. One of the main points of the program was to be able to detect exacerbation episodes in COPD patients. For this purpose, exacerbation was defined as an increase in dyspnoea along with two of the following criteria: increase in frequency of cough, increase in the amount of sputum, changes in the sputum color, or increase in ronchi.

Planned activities of the program included a monthly home visit by a skilled respiratory nurse under supervision of the physician, where the nurse provided the patient with verbal and written information on the disease, management of daily routine, exercise, understanding and use of drugs, health maintenance, and early recognition of signs that require medical intervention. When visiting patients, nurses applied a questionnaire including questions designed to detect changes in underlying respiratory symptoms regarding clinical symptoms associated with COPD exacerbation. When needed, a spirometry and an oximetry were also conducted during each home visit. The doctor was immediately informed if worsening was found in the clinical questionnaire or spirometry, or if there was a >2% drop in oxygen saturation with respect to hospital oximetry.

In addition to the home visits, the nurse telephoned the patient every 10 days to inquire about possible COPD symptoms associated with exacerbation, and the use of rescue medication. The frequency of telephone calls could be increased at the discretion of the nurse or physician. According to the symptoms reported by the patient, one of the following actions was taken: a home visit by a nurse, a visit to the hospital, or a telephone counseling followed a few days later by a control visit.

An analysis of the outcomes of this program showed that the HRQoL of COPD patients improved after implantation of our program and these changes were clinically relevant in several health dimensions. The analysis included the data collected for a period of 12 months after the implantation of the program. These data were compared with the data collected for 12 months previous to the implantation of the program. Pulmonary function data, gas exchange, and HRQoL were assessed before and after the implantation of the program. The HRQoL was assessed by the Medical Outcomes Study Short Form-36 (SF36) and the Saint George Respiratory Questionnaire (SGRQ). The study included 18 patients with COPD (16 men and 2 women) with a mean age of 69.4 ± 10.3 years and a body mass index of 26.6 ± 4.2 kg/m^2. All subjects had severe COPD and at least two hospital admissions for exacerbation in the previous year. We found significant improvements in the SGRQ total score (before: 42.5 ± 8.6; after: 35.5 ± 13.8; $p < 0.05$), activity (before: 14.9 ± 4.8; after: 11.2 ± 4.8; $p < 0.05$) and impact (before: 17.4 ± 4.6; after: 11.7 ± 4.5; $p < 0.05$) scores but not the symptom score (before: 12.6 ± 4.4; after: 13.6 ± 7.5; $p = $ns). In the SGRQ score system, the lower the value, the higher the improvement of the patient. With respect to SF36, significant improvement was found in mental health (before: 57.1 ± 20.0; after: 75.7 ± 9.2; $p < 0.05$) and energy/vitality dimensions (before: 46.5 ± 14.0; after: 54.7 ± 7.2; $p < 0.05$). In the SF36 score system, the higher the score, the higher the improvement.

Since our study showed that homecare for control of COPD patients had a significant positive impact, we started a second pilot project including 30 COPD patients. The goal of the project was that the patients could use IT to collect and transmit their own data to avoid the nurse visits. For this, PDA devices with communication capabilities (Bluetooth, GPRS/UMTS) were programmed to instruct the patients on how and when to collect the data (oximetry, electrocardiography, spirometry, and the questionnaires) and then transmit them to a server where it can be retrieved by a nurse or a physician. Data transmission between the clinical devices and PDAs is made via Bluetooth. In this setting, one of the main tasks of the nurses is to teach the patients how to use the PDA and the clinical devices. In this way, the nurse can be released from home visits still having control of the patients. An evaluation of this project is currently underway.

10.3
The Future of Telenursing for Respiratory Diseases

One of the most important future challenges facing health systems is the care of an increasing number of chronic patients. Among chronic conditions, COPD is particularly relevant because of its high prevalence. Patients with chronic pulmonary conditions may periodically present episodes of exacerbation that overload emergency departments with subsequently high cost for health systems. Currently, public health systems are oriented to acute phase treatment of illnesses and are not ready to properly address the needs of chronic patients.

The advances in IT make a new type of health management possible for patients with chronic respiratory diseases where the follow-up is relocated to their home in order to better anticipate potential exacerbation of their illness. In this setting, the nursing staff are prone to play a relevant role. Telenursing visits could substitute for a substantial fraction of on-site home nursing visits. This has important implications in terms of reducing the cost of home nursing care. In our experience, the nursing procedures can be effectively carried out by using IT as we showed telecare settings we have described.

Systems based on knowledge (SBK) represent a tool that may be useful for telenursing in the future. In recent years, a variety of approaches have appeared proposing the use of SBK for the purpose of analyzing increasingly abstract physiological data in conjunction with detailed clinical information to aid decision making. An SBK system could be suitable for monitoring patients with chronic respiratory diseases by means of telenursing procedures.

10.4
Summary

- Chronic respiratory diseases represent a major health-care problem for the public health-care systems. The new ways of delivering care remotely through telecare interventions may significantly contribute to solve this problem.
- The authors present three settings based on telecare procedures intended to deliver home health care to patients with chronic respiratory diseases, where the nursing staff plays a relevant role.
- Telenursing may reduce nurse home visits and can help keep a good control of patients with chronic respiratory diseases at home, which in turn would reduce hospital admissions and slow disease progression.

Acknowledgments This work was partially supported by grants BFU2007-61034 (MEC), BFU2010-14968 (MICINN), FEDER, NanoBioMed Consolider-Ingenio 2010, *Fondo Investigación Sanitaria* PI08/90769, and Rede Galega de Nanomedicina.

Glossary

Chronic obstructive pulmonary disease – A pulmonary condition caused by a combination of diseases including chronic bronchitis, emphysema, and chronic obstructive airways disease. The main symptom is an inability to breathe in and out properly.

Cost-effective – When related to health represents the relationship between a gain in health and the cost associated with the health gain.

Dyspnoea – Breathing discomfort. It is a common symptom of many medical disorders, particularly those related to the respiratory or cardiovascular systems.

Homecare – Health care or supportive care provided in the patient's home by health-care professionals.

Medical Outcomes Study Short Form-36 – A widely used, generic, patient-report measure created to assess health-related quality of life (HRQoL) in the general population.

Neuromuscular disease – A broad term that includes many diseases that involve muscle and/or nerves.

Oximetry – Monitoring the oxygenation of a patient's hemoglobin.

Oxygen saturation – The relative amount of oxygen that is carried in the blood.

Polygraph – Instrument that records several physiological events.

Polysomnography – A comprehensive recording of biomedical parameters during sleep.

Pulse oximeter – Medical device used to measure the oxygen saturation of a patient's blood.

Saint George Respiratory Questionnaire – A standardized self-completed questionnaire for measuring impaired health and perceived well-being ("quality of life") in airways disease.

Sleep apnea syndrome – A disorder characterized by pauses in breathing during sleep. In obstructive sleep apnea, breathing is interrupted by a physical block to airflow, despite the effort to breathe.

Sphygmomanometer – A device used to measure the blood pressure.

Spirometry – Measurement of the volume and/or glow of air that can be inhaled or exhaled. It is the most common pulmonary function test.

Systems based on knowledge – Intelligent tools working in a narrow domain to provide intelligent decisions with justification. Knowledge is acquired and represented using various knowledge representation techniques rules, frames, and scripts.

Telehealth – Delivery of health-related services by means of telecommunication technologies.

References

1. Bourbeau J, Julien M, Maltais F, et al. Reduction of hospital utilization in patients with chronic obstructive pulmonary disease. *Arch Intern Med*. 2003;163:585-591.
2. Bruderman I, Abboud S. Telespirometry: novel system for home monitoring of asthmatic patients. *Telemed J*. 1997;3:127-133.
3. De Lusignan S, Althans A, Wells S, et al. A pilot study of radiotelemetry for continuous cardiopulmonary monitoring of patients at home. *J Telemed Telecare*. 2000;6(Suppl 1):119-122.
4. Escourrou P, Luriau S, Rehel M, et al. Needs and costs of sleep monitoring. *Stud Health Technol Inform*. 2000;78:69-85.
5. Finkelstein SM, Lindgren B, Prasad B, et al. Reliability and validity of spirometry measurements in a paperless home monitoring diary program for lung transplantation. *Heart Lung*. 1993;22:523-533.
6. Gagnadoux F, Pelletier-Fleury N, Philippe C, et al. Home unattended vs hospital telemonitored polysomnography in suspected obstructive sleep apnea syndrome: a randomized crossover trial. *Chest*. 2002;121:753-758.
7. Global Initiative for Chronic Obstructive Lung Disease (GOLD). Global strategy for the diagnosis, management and prevention of COPD; 2006. Available from http://www.goldcopd.org
8. GOLD. The burden of lung disease, 2nd ed. A Statistics Report from the British Thoracic Society; 2006.
9. Gonzalez F, Iglesias R, Suarez A, et al. Teleophthalmology link between a primary health care center and a reference hospital. *Med Inform Internet Med*. 2001;26:251-263.
10. Hernandez C, Casas A, Escarrabill J, et al. Home hospitalisation of exacerbated chronic obstructive pulmonary disease patients. *Eur Respir J*. 2003;21:58-67.
11. Izbicki G, Abboud S. Telespirometry for home monitoring of pulmonary function. *J R Soc Med*. 1999;92:154-155.
12. Johns MW. A new method for measuring daytime sleepiness: the Epworth sleepiness scale. *Sleep*. 1991;14:540-545.
13. Johnston B, Wheeler L, Deuser J, et al. Outcomes of the Kaiser Permanente tele-home health research project. *Arch Fam Med*. 2000;9:40-45.
14. Kristo DA, Andrada T, Eliasson AH, et al. Telemedicine in the sleep laboratory: feasibility and economic advantages of polysomnograms transferred online. *Telemed J E Health*. 2001;7:219-224.
15. Kristo D, Eliasson AH, Netzer NC, et al. Application of telemedicine to sleep medicine. *Sleep Breath*. 2001;5:97-99.
16. Langsetmo L, Platt RW, Ernst P, et al. Under reporting exacerbation of chronic obstructive pulmonary disease in a longitudinal cohort. *Am J Respir Crit Care Med*. 2008;177:396-401.
17. Lee RG, Chen KC, Haiso C, et al. Mobile care system with an alert mechanism. *IEEE Trans Inf Technol Biomed*. 2007;11:507-517.
18. Mair FS, Wilkinson M, Bonnar SA, et al. The role of telecare in the management of exacerbations of chronic obstructive pulmonary disease in the home. *J Telemed Telecare*. 1999;5(Suppl 1):66-67.
19. McLean S, Sheikh A. Does telehealthcare offer a patient-centred way forward for the community-based management of long-term respiratory disease? *Prim Care Respir J*. 2009;18:125-126.
20. Mykytyn IJ, Sajkov D, Neill AM, et al. Portable computerized polysomnography in attended and unattended settings. *Chest*. 1999;115:114-122.
21. Pelletier-Fleury N, Gagnadoux F, Philippe C, et al. A cost-minimization study of telemedicine. The case of telemonitored polysomnography to diagnose obstructive sleep apnea syndrome. *Int J Technol Assess Health Care*. 2001;17:604-611.

22. Pelletier-Fleury N, Lanoe JL, Philippe C, et al. Economic studies and 'technical' evaluation of telemedicine: the case of telemonitored polysomnography. *Health Policy*. 1999;49:179-194.

23. Pinnock H, Slack R, Paglairi C, et al. Understanding the potential role of mobile phone-based monitoring and asthma self management of asthma: qualitative study. *Clin Exp Allergy*. 2007;37:794-802.

24. Rodriguez De Castro C, Ordonez AJ, Navarrete P, et al. Usefulness of telemedicine in chronic diseases: home tele-care of patient with chronic obstructive pulmonary disease. *Med Clin (Barc)*. 2002;119:301-303.

25. Skwarska E, Cohen G, Skwarski KM, et al. Randomised controlled trial of supported discharge in patients with exacerbations of chronic obstructive pulmonary disease. *Thorax*. 2002;55:907-912.

26. Vontetsianos T, Giovas P, Katsaras T, et al. Telemedicine-assisted home support for patients with advanced chronic obstructive pulmonary disease: preliminary results after nine-month follow-up. *J Telemed Telecare*. 2005;11(Suppl 1):86-88.

27. Wilkinson T, Donaldson GC, Hurst JR, et al. Early therapy improves outcomes of exacerbations of chronic obstructive pulmonary disease. *Am J Respir Crit Care Med*. 2004;169:1298-1303.

28. Zamarrón C, Gude F, Barcala J, et al. Utility of oxygen saturation and heart rate spectral analysis obtained from pulse oximetric recordings in the diagnosis of sleep apnea syndrome. *Chest*. 2003;123:1567-1576.

Telenursing in Africa

11

Sinclair Wynchank and Jill Fortuin

Abbreviations

AIDS	Acquired Immune Deficiency Syndrome
ECG	Electrocardiography
HCW	Health-care Worker
HIV	Human Immunodeficiency Virus
ICT	Information and Computer Technology
NEPAD	New Partnership for African Development
PHC	Primary Health care
RN	State Registered Nurse
SADC	Southern African Development Community
TB	Tuberculosis
WHO	World Health Organisation

11.1
Introduction

Nursing is a caring profession. Lay persons think of a nurse taking care of the sick and aiding normal development in the young. But nursing is much more than this and telenursing efficiently promotes and supports aspects of all nursing activities. Telenursing has various definitions. All of them incorporate an electronic transfer of information relevant to nursing and use information and computer technology (ICT). Telenursing can pass

J. Fortuin (✉)
Telemedicine Platform, Medical Research Council, Tygerberg 7505, 19070, Cape Town, South Africa
e-mail: jill.fortuin@mrc.ac.za

S. Kumar and H. Snooks (eds.), *Telenursing*, Health Informatics,
DOI: 10.1007/978-0-85729-529-3_11, © Springer-Verlag London Limited 2011

knowledge (e.g., to aid in the management of a patient or assist distance-learning/ professional development) and serve the other activities of a nurse. We consider a nurse as a person who has been trained to care for the sick, infirm, and disabled, and who promotes health, healthy growth, and development in children and others. African telenursing is in its infancy and is currently establishing its own norms and practices. Over a hundred times as much has been published on telenursing, from developed nations, compared with developing countries. This is because telenursing was first introduced into technically advanced nations. There it was refined, taking advantage of improvements in relevant technology. At the same time its applications were steadily extended and only then was there growing use of telenursing in developing countries. In this way telenursing has followed the progress of telemedicine. Sufficient progress has been made so it is now appropriate to review telenursing in Africa, especially in its developing nations. Viewing it from South Africa is especially opportune for several reasons. Many millions of South Africans have socioeconomic circumstances typical of the developing world. But there are also technology, health care, and infrastructure in parts of South Africa, characteristic of developed nations. Since 1994, when South Africa became democratic, there has been greatly increasing cooperation with less-developed African countries. Many joint health programs are now underway and transfer of telenursing activity, mentioned above, from developed to developing countries, is now taking place between South Africa and other African states. Understanding telenursing's achievements elsewhere can aid this transfer and the establishment of telenursing in Africa. Such study will prevent unnecessary duplication of existing equipment and methods, while allowing appropriate modification of existing telenursing for African needs.

Africa lacks health-care workers (HCWs), with 4.3 million needed worldwide. The greatest needs are in the poorest nations, where nurses form the backbone of public health-care systems. This is especially true in sub-Saharan Africa.[25] Rural, periurban, and urban nurse-directed clinics have played a crucial role in South African public health, where the nursing staff have much responsibility and independence. Few studies have been made of patients' attitudes to the health care they receive from nurses in developing countries. But such nurse-practitioners, the concept of which was first introduced into the USA in 1965, are now known there by 90% of the population. Their services have been used by about 60% of American residents and 82% of them have been satisfied, or very satisfied, with this nursing care.[3] It is likely that such percentages will be even greater in Africa, where alternative health care is often less readily available. Telenursing can support acquisition and maintenance of these high levels of responsibility and independence. Also it helps in the provision of the necessary teaching with the existing distance-learning programs, described below. Studies by the WHO and others[33] of health workforce needs have been made for Ethiopia, Ghana, Kenya, Malawi, Tanzania, and other developing countries. Suggested ways to supply requirements include increased use of ICTs and modular education. Telenursing is intimately involved in both. In Ethiopia, which is typical of developing Africa, 60–80% of health problems are due to largely preventable communicable diseases, such as malaria, pneumonia, viral infections, and TB.[5] Here too telenursing can play a part in relevant education. HIV/AIDS is a serious danger to the health of Africans and nurse-directed primary health care (PHC) clinics throughout Africa have a crucial role in combating this pandemic. Telenursing is already recognized and in use as an extensive and effective means of disseminating information and knowledge in the fight against this scourge.

11.2
Setting Up Telenursing

Careful thought and preparation must be given to the preparation for telenursing activity, especially in Africa, where a simple reproduction of an existing service elsewhere is usually totally unsuitable. Funds generally lack in all developing countries, so extensive modifications or duplications will be unaffordable. It is not sufficient to buy equipment, combine it with a telecommunication system, and then go ahead.[36] Dedicated involvement of local leaders and medical bodies is essential and in each country relevant economic and cultural principles must be considered. Also governmental support should always be sought, especially for questions regarding regulation and to help smooth integration with existing services.[38] Suitable technology must be identified, after considering available infrastructure, local users' levels of computer literacy, etc. It must be appreciated that telenursing is not a panacea for all nursing problems and activities. A recent study in South Africa found that because of the lack of coordination between health services of the nine provinces there is no single ICT system available to be deployed throughout the country to assist in the struggle against HIV/AIDS.[29] All these reemphasize the need for adequate preparation before embarking on a widely based telenursing service. In the later stages of planning, and after some hands-on experience, nurse-users should be encouraged to suggest changes in equipment and procedures. This may improve "device-friendliness" and its effective application.[14] Such an approach allowed a simple, ruggedized telenursing workstation devised in South Africa to provide modified menus and a remote control. This made its application less frightening for nurses with little or no previous ICT experience. Some of Africa's poorest households are located in regions with good mobile phone signals and there has been an unexpectedly rapid uptake of mobile telephony in all levels of African society. This may be incorporated into aspects of telenursing as has been done in India.[21] Its value has already been demonstrated as having been very useful in the UK for various serious chronic conditions.[2] Using this type of communication to ensure wise use in medical emergencies would be a practical and simple introduction of such technology in Africa.[4] Challenges to nursing in the twenty-first century must be overcome. These challenges include nursing shortages and maldistribution, consequent negative affectivity, increasingly complex clinical practice, and changing nursing service delivery systems. To defeat them, aids, such as information, instruction and mentorship to help nurses in isolated locations, can be effectively delivered by telenursing.[10] Software used in telenursing triage recommendations has been evaluated and was found to be more useful for assessment than decision making. It had limitations in providing information and supporting learning and overemphasized acute conditions.[16] So, such software if used in Africa should be appropriately modified.

11.3
Telenursing Experience and Application

Although most telenursing activities originated in developed nations, steady application to Africa continues and a variety of projects is underway. A representative selection is outlined in this chapter. Many of the lessons already learned are applied, as telenursing becomes more established in Africa and as African levels of computer experience and infrastructure increase. The only nursing database in a sub-Saharan African developing nation has been set up in Kenya.[27] It provides reliable nursing information about workforce capacity, demographics, and migration patterns, thus allowing assistance in determining optimum use of health personnel. A project to aid Zambian nurses infected and affected by HIV/AIDS has determined that a focus on appropriate training, monitoring, and setting up of local support groups can significantly improve their situation.[31] The tele-education aspect of this focus permits a telenursing approach, which will allow a more extensive teaching at reduced cost, compared with traditional methods. There are established WHO guidelines for the feeding of infants of HIV-infected mothers to prevent mother-to-child transmission of the virus. Although three clear criteria have been established, almost 70% of HIV-infected mothers in South Africa were found to be unable to fulfill these criteria. Their feeding methods give an increased risk of HIV transmission and death to their infants. Counseling of these mothers is urgently required, in many African nations, in addition to South Africa. Guidelines for nurses in PHC clinics to counsel and train counselors can efficiently be disseminated by telenursing distance-learning.[9] Another important aspect of the HIV/AIDS pandemic in Africa is the resulting stigma suffered by those infected. This stigma has been clearly shown to violate human rights in Lesotho, Malawi, South Africa, Swaziland, and Tanzania, where a broad investigation was done.[22] Further, many believe that until this stigma is conquered the illness will not be fully defeated. About 5% of the world's adults have diabetes mellitus and its incidence in developing countries is steadily growing. It has well-known, serious complications, including blindness, stroke, and cardiovascular disease, particularly in developing countries.[24] Nurses are in the frontline in ensuring that its sufferers become able to manage their condition and a telephonic telenursing has been shown to be effective in doing so for African-American women in the USA.[1] Attempts to extend this to Africa are underway. One lead ECG signals are particularly suited for low-technology-based telenursing and their use in nurse triage has been demonstrated as most appropriate in chronic heart failure.[17] An ongoing telenursing project aiding isolated chronically ill rural women in five states of the USA has found that a nurse-directed computer-based health support system had better health outcomes than face-to-face contact.[32] Its participants exerted greater efforts to improve functioning, demonstrated greater resistance to psychological illness, and improved ability to self-manage their chronic condition.[28] The nurse monitor was a facilitator, not effector.[32] She/he watched daily exchanges, for inappropriateness, health-threatening advice, suicidal tendencies, etc., and made personal contact if required. Each participant (with minimal ICT background) needed access to a computer and needed to be able to use English. Although this project may be thought inappropriate to include when considering African telenursing, it does indicate a successful future application, for the WHO has identified chronic illness as the major health burden globally[35] and, with the steadily increasing use of telenursing, such activity is likely to achieve importance in Africa's mid-term future.

11.4
Education and Training Opportunities

What must a telenurse know and do? She/he must be a fully qualified state registered nurse (RN) and when in direct contact with a caller she/he must be able to assess, refer, advise, support, strengthen, and teach and facilitate a caller's learning, as necessary, offering triage and self-care advice if required.[20] So, for this, telenurses need high levels of competence. Already one authority, the Queensland State Government, in Australia, has introduced the formal qualification of "telenurse." This requires an RN to undergo further study and training.[26] Since most telenurses and callers for telephonic nursing are female, gender plays an important role in telenursing. In Africa, and in many other societies, telenurses need training in handling overt or covert power messages based on supposed male superiority and their training must recognize this.[15]

Distance-learning is an integral part of telenursing and its suitable application can provide knowledge for telenursing and/or other nursing activity. Already tele-education projects to aid telenursing have been set up in African and other developing countries. In Eritrea, there is a distance-learning project set up in association with a USA group for RNs to study advanced nursing practice and possibly be prepared to teach in nursing colleges.[19] The initial subject chosen was midwifery. Lessons learned to ensure success include use of relevant technology, adequate preparation for participants, an emphasis on clinical education, and allowing flexibility in the material presented, after input from the students. A South African project serving a large nurse-run clinic set up an audiovisual telenursing link between the Department of Psychology of the University of the Western Cape and the PHC clinic, 450 km away. The clinic's mental health service is supervised by this department. Since the two institutions are so far apart, little in-person supervision is possible. The link allowed assessment when agitated patients presented, especially at weekends. Otherwise, they would be taken to local police cells till a district surgeon made a visit on the following Monday. The link was also used for teaching purposes on the campus, when patients whose pathology was rarely encountered in the department's urban setting were encountered. Since such links are bidirectional, distance-learning techniques were also used to train two types of lay-counselor in the clinic's catchment area, where there is much domestic and other violence and also a high incidence of substance abuse, alcoholism, and the fetal alcohol syndrome. These volunteer lay-counselors were either professional persons (clergymen, librarians, nurses, teachers, social workers, etc.) or senior high-school students, and each group trained separately. The latter were particularly effective in counseling fellow learners. Regrettably, this successful program ended prematurely after theft of the equipment. Although childhood mortality has decreased in recent years, neonatal mortality has stayed constant or has increased in many developing countries. The majority of these deaths occur in the first 7 days and of them 70% are preventable. The WHO, UNICEF, and others have jointly addressed this problem and an "essential newborn care program" to combat it has been derived and evaluated in Zambia.[3] A self-directed computer-controlled course was found to be as successful in improving knowledge as a traditional hands-on-training version in studies undertaken in Zambia and South Africa.[23] The former is much less expensive and this is critical in resource-limited countries. Other telenursing programs will perform such evaluations and are likely to follow a similar route. It is well known that in Africa malaria is a major cause of morbidity and mortality. About 90% of life-threatening malaria occurs in children with highest mortality for those under 5 years. An assessment was made in Malawi of the clinical care underway in many parts of the developing world, to determine areas of improvement in malaria management.[8] It was found that modified care was required at the first referral level. Ways of disseminating and implementing these findings should be by means of telenursing to inform PHC clinics in all affected African countries.

Telenursing programs in resource-rich nations can often be applied, after modification, for local specific needs, milieu and infrastructure, in developing countries. Examples of such existing programs, useful for African application, follow. Nurses are most prominent in disaster-stricken areas as suppliers of health care. So, a UK-derived postgraduate quali-fication in disaster relief nursing uses a tele-education strategy. It underlines effective use of transcultural nursing and is appropriate for use in many developing countries.[6] A nurse-led web-based pilot coaching program in the Netherlands has helped high-risk patients to change their vascular risk profile, by improving their ability to self-manage.[11] This princi-ple too will be suitable for African application. Pediatric resuscitation knowledge and facilities frequently lack in developing countries. An initial attempt to correct this resulted in training in Australia of Vietnamese nurses, who had a wide range of backgrounds, and others.[37] Inclusion of nations from Africa in such programs and provision of updates of relevant information can effectively use telenursing principles.

A practical way of making distance-learning easily available is to set up a web-based program. Many web-based distance-learning nursing programs have been set up, usually in resource-rich countries. This mode is slowly being introduced into other countries. Some examples of existing African nursing projects, partially or mainly web based, fol-low. Palliative care is often a field where nurses predominate. In Africa, the only formal qualifications in this area (a diploma and M.Phil.) are offered by the University of Cape Town, South Africa. Since the course began in 2001, 172 students have registered for it and the course almost entirely depends on tele-education techniques, with suitably restricted web-based access to the teaching material. Students must be postgraduate nurses or doctors. The course's curriculum is suitable for local conditions and the material taught emphasizes family dynamics in the extended and nonnuclear family (this is particularly relevant to HIV/AIDS) and palliative care and bereavement in children. So far, students have come from 12 anglophone African countries. The course's importance is underlined by the realization that some of the continent's nations currently have no expertise in pallia-tive care. There is an increasing need for such skills to manage current levels of HIV/AIDS and other highly prevalent serious conditions (E. Gwyther, 2009, personal communica-tion). This successful program will be followed in 2010 by another tele-education M.Phil. course in public mental health from the same university. It is also available to postgraduate nurses and initially will emphasize policy planning and implementation (A. Flisher, 2009, personal communication) A pediatric oncology – hematology web-base program serves nurses in Morocco and other developing countries.[34] Its importance reflects the facts that overall pediatric cancer cure rates are about 75% in developed countries and a third of this in developing nations, where it can be the leading cause of death in children aged 5–15 years. But about 80–85% of all childhood cancers occur in developing countries, where survival can be under 10%.[7] A further application of a web-based site has been for a nursing study in Ethiopia and other developing countries studying a mother's mental health and her child's nutrition status. This work "confirms that promotion of maternal mental health may be important for the improvement of child nutrition."[12] Obstetric complications are a frequent cause of death in developing countries and worldwide this causes <500,000 deaths yearly.[18] The assessment and improving of skilled birth attendants in Benin, Rwanda, and other developing countries has recently been underway, with WHO support. A website played an important role in training local assessors and this successful pilot scheme has been extended to Niger and Kenya.[13]

11.5
Ethical Questions in Telenursing

Nursing ethics is a much studied field and telenursing introduces additional challenging ethical considerations, which so far have received little attention. Also many of the ethical problems of traditional hands-on nursing apply to telenursing. A Swedish study of telenursing's ethical dilemmas[17] applies to Africa. Documentation associated with telephonic telenursing is especially sensitive, if the nurse cannot be fully certain of the caller's identity. Other difficulties, frequently experienced in South Africa, and other multicultural societies, arise from discussion of personal and sensitive problems when the nurse and patient are members of different cultures. The patient's cultural tradition must be respected at all times, even if it contributes to problems in communication and if the nurse and patient have different norms concerning gender, etc., in society. As a consequence, the nurse may feel that her/his autonomy is compromised. Another ethical difficulty can arise for nurses when standardized protocols advise one type of action, but intuition and/or experience and/or knowledge prompt the nurse to believe that something else is more appropriate. In Africa, there is frequently a lack of resources and the health-care system's organization often prevents the telenurse from acting in what she/he believes to be the best interest of the caller. Preliminary work suggests that it will be necessary to explore differences in ethical dilemmas experienced by female and male nurses, for the two genders differ in their moral reasoning and possibly in other ways, which may affect their function as telenurses.[39] Nurse training should include appropriate ethical material, but for telenurses the necessary additional ethical features must be included.

11.6
Discussion

In Africa, telenursing is poised to become an important aid to the provision of improved health care and those pilots, and other, telenursing schemes underway and described above, bear this out. In South Africa, the basic nursing curriculum now includes material on ICT and those nurse-practitioners (typically in remote rural nurse-directed clinics) who practice telenursing should receive additional instruction. A resulting benefit of telenursing is that, after referring several patients with comparable problems, a nurse-practitioner often becomes able to manage similar patients without consultation. This is well demonstrated in a South African pilot teledermatology program. In it nurses often refer patients who finally prove to be HIV positive, for over 95% of HIV-infected patients have dermatological problems and their severity closely mirrors the infection's progress. As the nurses received telediagnoses and suggested management regimes through the telenursing link, they gained experience and confidence. Gradually, they were referring fewer HIV-positive patients with skin lesions, for they had learned how to diagnose and manage them locally. Apart from such practical learning, telenursing brings other benefits in South Africa. All telenursing links are two way and so formal education programs can be sent to the remote clinics, in addition to the links providing expert advice for specific nursing problems. The University of Cape Town has devised a series of 14 computer-controlled modular distance-learning programs on aspects of community pediatrics. These are freely available for nurses in rural community health centers and clinics, who often have no regular direct access to pediatricians (M. Kibel, 2009, personal communication). Other tele-education in different nursing fields are also available and/or under development. In South Africa, there is compulsory community service of 1 year for newly graduated nurses, who are usually assigned to remote rural areas where there is the greatest lack of HCWs. In spite of working with experienced colleagues, they frequently feel very isolated. With telenursing facilities at their workplace their sense of isolation is greatly reduced, leading to a happier and more productive community service. These benefits of telenursing are available in South Africa, but they are slowly being extended to other African countries through regional collaborations. Initially, South Africa's inter-African projects are with 15 regional states through SADC (Southern African Development Community). However, plans are advanced for collaborations with more distant African nations, through NEPAD (New Partnership for African Development), which comprises 18 countries throughout entire Africa. Both these organizations have emphasized health aspects of inter-African nation cooperation and development. So the pilot and other telenursing activities underway in South Africa are steadily being extended beyond its borders. Very few costing studies of telenursing have been reported, but in developed countries there are clear cost benefits, especially from reduction in travel. Another great benefit of telenursing is improved local care, resulting from experience directly gained from the telenursing links, as described above. Also there are the benefits of tele-education. This allows more cost-effective provision of many forms of continuing nursing education, since travel costs are very greatly reduced for pupils and/or teachers. But it must not be forgotten that a crucial benefit of telenursing is the provision of improved service, especially for those in remote areas. Telenursing may even cost more than the traditional service it supplements (which could be no service at all), but the improvement can be so great that overall it is far preferable. In this way a distant but attainable goal for African telenursing is for all Africans to have free continuous telephonic access to telenursing advice and symptom triage, as is so for most Australians and all New Zealand residents.[30]

11.7
Conclusions

Africa's telenursing in its infancy and has absorbed lessons learned from telenursing else-where, its techniques and equipment, all of which are being applied and modified for the African situation and programs. Both collaborative telenursing programs with resource-rich nations and purely African telenursing are underway. Telenursing has already proved its value in pilot schemes and is ready to be extended to more nations in the continent.

11.8
Summary

The important points discussed in this chapter include the following:

- The nursing profession and telenursing
- Africa's health priorities
- Setting up telenursing in Africa
- African telenursing projects
- Web-based telenursing
- Telenursing and ethics
- African nursing education underway with telenursing

Acknowledgments   The authors wish to thank Ashley Bess for valuable administrative assis-tance and also Professors A. Flisher, E. Gwyther, and M. Kibel for informative discussions.

Glossary

Distance-learning – An education system that does not depend on teacher and learner being at the same place at the same time. Communication between them is usually by electronic means.

Ethics – Study of conduct and judgments using moral principles.

Palliative care – Managing a health condition to reduce severity of symptoms and/or improve quality of life. It does not try to cure or otherwise affect the condition and is usu-ally associated with a terminal situation, such as found in some cancers.

Tele-education – As for distance-learning.

Telenursing – An electronic transfer of information to aid a nursing activity.

Web-based – A system of making information available that operates over the Internet.

Website – One or more documents available through the Internet.

References

1. Amoako E, Skelly AH, Rossen EK. Outcomes of an intervention to reduce uncertainty among African American women with diabetes. *West J Nurs Res.* 2008;30(8):928-942. Epub 2 July 2008.
2. Blake H. Mobile phone technology in chronic disease management. *Nurs Stand.* 2008;23(12): 43-46.
3. Brown DJ. Consumers perspectives on nurse practitioners and independent practice. *J Am Acad Nurse Pract.* 2007;19(10):523-529.
4. Byass P, D'Ambruoso L. Cellular telephone networks in developing countries. *Lancet.* 2008;371(9613):650.
5. Crisp N, Gawanas B, Sharp I. Training the health workforce: scaling up, saving lives. *Lancet.* 2008;371(9613):689-691.
6. Davies K, Deeny P, Raikkonen M. A transcultural ethos underpinning curriculum development: a master's programme in disaster relief nursing. *J Transcult Nurs.* 2003;14(4): 349-357.
7. Day SW, Dycus PM, Chismark EA, et al. Quality assessment of paediatric oncology nursing in a Central American country: findings, recommendations, and preliminary outcomes. *Pediatr Nurs.* 2008;34(5):367-373.
8. Diep PP, Lien L, Hofman J. A criteria-based clinical audit on the case-management of children presenting with malaria at Mangochi District Hospital, Malawi. *World Hosp Health Serv.* 2007;43(2):21-29.
9. Doherty T, Chopra M, Jackson D, et al. Effectiveness of the WHO/UNICEF guidelines on infant feeding for HIV-positive women: results from a prospective cohort study in South Africa. *AIDS.* 2007;21(13):1791-1797.
10. Donley R. Challenges for nursing in the 21st century. *Nurs Econ.* 2005;23(6):312-318. 279.
11. Goessens BM, Visseren FL, de Nooijer J, et al. A pilot-study to identify the feasibility of an internet-based coaching programme for changing the vascular risk profile of high-risk patients. *Patient Educ Couns.* 2008;73(1):67-72. Epub 18 July 2008.
12. Harpham T, Huttly S, De Silva MJ, et al. Maternal mental health and child nutritional status in four developing countries. *J Epidemiol Community Health.* 2005;56(12):1060-1064.
13. Harvey SA, Blandon YC, McCaw-Binns A, et al. Are skilled birth attendants really skilled? A measurement method, some disturbing results and a potential way forward. *Bull World Health Organ.* 2007;85(10):783.
14. Hibbert D, Mair FS, Angus RM, et al. Lessons from the implementation of a home telecare service. *J Telemed Telecare.* 2003;9(Suppl 1):S55-S56.
15. Hoglung AT, Holmstrom I. It's easier to talk to a woman. Aspects of gender in Swedish telenursing. *J Clin Nurs.* 2008;17(22):2979-2986.
16. Holmstrom I. Decision aid software programs in telenursing: not used as intended? Experiences of Swedish telenursing. *Nurs Health Sci.* 2007;9(1):23-28.
17. Holmstrom I, Hoglung AT. The faceless encounter: ethical dilemmas in telephone nursing. *J Clin Nurs.* 2007;16(10):1865-1871.
18. Islam M. The safe motherhood initiative and beyond. *Bull World Health Organ.* 2007;85:735.
19. Johnson P, Ghebreyohanes V, Kutenplon D, et al. Distance education to prepare nursing faculty in Eritrea: diffusion of an innovative model of midwifery education. *J Midwifery Womens Health.* 2007;2(5):e37-e41.
20. Kaminsky E, Rosenqvist U, Holmstrom I. Telenurses' understanding of work: detective or educator? *J Adv Nurs.* 2009;65(2):382-390. Epub 27 November 2008.

21. Kanthraj GR, Srinivas CR. Store and forward teledermatology. *Indian J Dermatol Venereol Leprol*. 2007;73(1):5-12.
22. Kohi TW, Makoae L, Chirwa M, et al. HIV and AIDS stigma violates human rights in five African countries. *Nurs Ethics*. 2006;13(4):404-415.
23. McClure EM, Carlo WA, Wright LL, et al. Evaluation of the educational impact of the WHO essential newborn care course in Zambia. *Acta Paediatr*. 2007;96(8):1135-1138. Epub 3 July 2007.
24. Meetoo D, McGovern P, Safadi R. An epidemiological overview of diabetes across the world. *Br J Nurs*. 2007;16(16):1002-1007.
25. Ogilvie L, Mill JE, Astle B, et al. The exodus of health professionals from sub-Saharan Africa: balancing human rights and societal needs in the twenty-first century. *Nurs Inq*. 2007;14(2):114-124.
26. Anonymous, "Professional qualification of 'telenurse' (Queensland, Australia)", 2009 from website: http://www.health.qld.gov.au/workforus/careers/Telenurse.pdf
27. Riley P, Vindigni SM, Waudo AN, et al. Developing a nursing database system in Kenya. *Health Serv Res*. 2007;42(3 Pt 2):1389-1405.
28. Snooks HA, Williams AM, Griffiths LJ, et al. Real nursing? The development of telenursing. *J Adv Nurs*. 2008;61(6):631-640.
29. Sorenson T, Ulrike R, Fortuin J. A review of ICT-systems for HIV/AIDS and anti-retroviral treatment management in South Africa. *J Telemed Telecare*. 2008;14(1):37-41. review.
30. St George I, Cullen M, Gardiner L, et al. Universal telenursing triage in Australia and New Zealand – a new primary healthcare service. *Aust Fam Physician*. 2008;37(6):476-479.
31. Vitols MP, du Plessis E, Ng'andu O. Mitigating the plight of HIV-infected and affected nurses in Zambia. *Int Nurs Rev*. 2007;54(4):375-382.
32. Weinert C, Cudney S, Winters C. Social support in cyberspace: the next generation. *Comput Inform Nurs*. 2005;23(1):7-15.
33. WHO. *World Health Report 2006: Working Together for Health*. Geneva: World Health Organization; 2006.
34. Williams JA, Ribeiro RC. Pediatric hematology – oncology outreach for developing countries. *Hematol Oncol Clin North Am*. 2001;15(4):775-787. x.
35. Le Gales-Camus C, Beaglehole R, Epping-Jordan JA, et al. Preventing chronic diseases: a vital investment: WHO global report, Geneva; 2005. ISBN 92 4 156300 1.
36. Yellowlees P. How not to develop telemedicine systems. *Telemed Today*. 1997;5(3):6-7. 17.
37. Young S, Hutchinson A, Nguyen VT, et al. Teaching paediatric resuscitation skills in developing country: introduction of the advanced paediatric life support course in Vietnam. *Emerg Med Australas*. 2008;20(3):271-275.
38. Yun EK, Park HA. Factors affecting the implementation of telenursing in Korea. *Stud Health Technol Inform*. 2006;122:657-659.
39. Zickmund S. Care and justice: the impact of gender and profession on ethical decision making in the healthcare arena. *J Clin Ethics*. 2004;15:176-187.

Telenursing in Sweden

12

Inger Holmström

Abbreviations

CDSS	Computerized Decision Support System
ECTS	European Credit Transfer System (1.5 ECTS is equivalent to 1 week studies)
GP	General Practitioner
ICN	International Council of Nurses
IT	Information Technology
SHD	Swedish Healthcare Direct

12.1
Background/Setting

12.1.1
Setting/Brief Description of Health-Care System

The number of call centers staffed with telenurses in Sweden has rapidly increased during the last decade, as well as the number of calls per center.[24] Telenursing is, although more and more centralized, a diversified activity in Sweden, based on, e.g., geographical conditions and the population in the local area. The Swedish health-care system is tax financed and private health-care providers are still rare outside the larger cities. There is a strong emphasis on equal health care for all within the Swedish health-care system, established in the Swedish Health and Medical Service Act (1982:763). Sweden has a decentralized health-care system where services to a large extent are based on decisions made by local politicians in the 20 counties. The citizens pay taxes to local authorities, which have a great deal of freedom to organize health-care services in their area.

I. Holmström
Department of Public Health and Caring Sciences, Uppsala University, Health Services
Research, SE-751 22, Box 564, Uppsala, Sweden
e-mail: inger.holmstrom@pubcare.uu.se

S. Kumar and H. Snooks (eds.), *Telenursing*, Health Informatics,
DOI: 10.1007/978-0-85729-529-3_12, © Springer-Verlag London Limited 2011

A national project for the development of telenursing started in 1997. However, telenursing call centers did not emerge on a broad scale until 2000–2001. The national telenursing helpline is labeled Swedish Healthcare Direct (SHD). Some reasons for the development of telenursing call centers were high costs for medical care, long waiting times for doctor's appointments, and distance to family, who traditionally had given advice when nearby.[25] Furthermore, politicians had, and still have, a wish to make health service and medical care more efficient by steering flows of patients[20] to appropriate level of care. Efficient telephone advice nursing is one way of managing limited resources in health care. Telenursing in Sweden has been shown to be cost-effective and time saving and to increase patient self-care ability.[16] Furthermore, it provides an opportunity for health promotion.

During the 1990s, the Swedish health-care system underwent major structural changes and financial cutbacks. These financial cutbacks resulted in staff reduction, and increased distress and work-load among staff.[2] In addition, many Swedish nurses will retire during the next decade creating a situation when there is a lack of experienced nurses. At the same time, the numbers of old and very old people will rise. This situation is a challenge for society, the health-care organization, and professionals. Furthermore, Sweden is currently a multicultural society, which also creates new demands on the health-care sector.

12.1.2
Nursing Education and Practice in Sweden

Swedish nursing education consists of a 3-year program with admission requirements similar to other university programs. Applicants must have completed general upper secondary school. The program is comprised of theoretical and clinical courses. Approximately 40% of the nursing education consists of clinical practice. After gaining some work experience the nurses can join specialist nurse education within different fields, such as intensive care or pediatrics (year-long courses) or midwifery education (18-month course). These courses are needed for positions in specialized care or independent and supervisory functions. There is, however, no one single education for telenurses in Sweden. Hence, telenurses have a variety of specialist nursing backgrounds, such as district nursing, acute and emergency care nursing, or pediatric nursing. However, there is a current discussion about the need for a formal telenursing university course, aimed at providing a solid practice for telenurses and, furthermore, to ensure that telenursing gets the same status as other nursing specialties. The Swedish nursing workforce consists of about 90% females.

Telenurses should in most cases be the first contact when the public want to get in contact with the health-care system, especially during out-of-hours. The Swedish nurses independently assess, triage, and give self-care advice; refer the caller to an appropriate level of care; or book an appointment with the general practitioner (GP) on call.[25] The organization of telenursing in Sweden is very flat indeed because it consists of only two levels: managers and telenurses. Hence, there are no call-handlers or receptionists employed at SHD. According to Valsecchi et al.[23] the Swedish telenurses are far more autonomous compared to their British colleagues, but they also have more responsibilities. Hence, they are more vulnerable but have a stronger professionalism.

The working environment at the national telenursing helpline SHD is in many ways comparable to any other call center, with high demands of efficiency from the employer.

Swedish telenurses feel conflicting demands of being both carer and gatekeeper.[10] Callers want and need time to describe their complaints and nurses are trained to care for patients as unique individuals with differing needs. However, the expectations are that average calls should be about 6–8 min. Telenurses are also well aware that telephone queues make callers annoyed and dissatisfied.[26]

12.1.3
Telecommunication and Other Relevant Infrastructure

As early as in the 1930s, patients in Sweden started to consult nurses by telephone, often to get a doctor's appointment. During the 1990s, the Swedish health-care system changed and telenurses were given a more distinct role. Currently, the number of calls as well as the number of inhabitants who can reach a telenurse at SHD by its telephone number 1177 is, as stated above, rapidly increasing. At the end of 2009, 8 million of about 9.5 million Swedes are estimated to have access to SHD. SHD strives to create opportunities for a telenursing network with possibilities to achieve both local and national advantages. The explicit goals are as follows: increased safety for the public, improved access to competent telenurses and their advice, and also improved efficiency. This could lead to better and more effective use of resources when the number of unnecessary doctors' appointments or care at too high a care level could be reduced or avoided. Hence, there are considerable demands on telenurses. The SHD is very similar to NHS Direct in the UK and Health Direct in Western Australia. Compared to, for example, NHS Direct in Great Britain, Swedish call centers included in the network SHD are less centralized and combine both public and private delivery.[23]

SHD is also accessible online (http://www.sjukvardsradgivning.se/). The website 1177. se provides reliable information and easy-access services within the health-care area. It is intended to enhance health among the public, strengthen the patients' position, be a part of the health-care sector, and work without commercial interest (accessed January 12, 2010). The website is owned by all county councils and provided free of charge. The texts are written by physicians, nurses, dentists, pharmacists, and other professionals. These texts are regularly updated. The website 1177.se contains numerous facts and advice about illnesses, injuries, and symptoms such as:

- Examinations, treatments and medications
- Pregnancy, delivery, parenthood, and child health care
- Health promotion and well-being
- Crises and difficulties in life
- The healthy body and how it works
- Rights and obligations for patients and health-care professionals
- Facilities for disabled

For small children there is a special part of the site called Kids Department. On this part of the site cartoon movies are shown. In a playful and educational manner, these movies are thought to prepare children for treatments and examinations in health care and during hospitalization.

1177 self-care guide ("Egenvårdsguiden") is a book with hands-on self-care advice from the web page. The content of the book is also accessible online. *1177 self-care guide* contains hundreds of suggestions and pieces of advice about how to proceed to manage common simple symptoms by self-care. There is also help to make judgments about when to contact the health-care services for a professional assessment. Many county councils offer their inhabitants the book free of charge.

12.2
Current Telenursing Practice

12.2.1
General Statistics: Extent of Telenursing

As described above, Swedish telenursing has currently entered a centralization strategy but is adapted to local practices in each county. At this stage, the end of 2009, only 3 out of 20 county councils have not joined the network (Ferm I., 2009, Personal Communication). The counties that join the telephone network receive a total system solution consisting of telephone equipment, electronic documentation, and computerized decision support system (CDSS). The telephone equipment contains a telephone queue system that is able to integrate different counties during periods of high demand in a given county. The system also generates statistics about number of calls answered, length of the calls, and queue situation. The calls are often tape-recorded.

Currently, about 800 telenurses are working within the SHD network (Ferm I., 2009, Personal Communication). The telenursing services are provided by registered nurses at SHD, but also at specialized departments such as pediatric clinics and health-care centers, and by the alarm number 112 for emergency issues. (The calls to the alarm number 112 are handled by call handlers, who can consult a nurse if they feel the need for higher medical competency.) In 2006, 33% of Swedish inhabitants called the health-care services for advice.[21] At the telenursing call centers most calls are received during morning and evening hours at weekends (Jansson G., 2007, Written report supplied by Gunilla Jansson, Unpublished). The most common reasons for calling are infections such as fever or sore throat.[27] About 33% of the calls are made by a third party. Calls about sick children vary between 30% and 40% in different parts of Sweden.[12] About 65% of callers are female[14] and they seem to call not only for themselves, but also for children, friends, and relatives. Telenurses express that they find it easier to talk to female callers and that female callers are more easily persuaded to wait and see compared to male callers who are experienced as more assertive and demanding.[8] Telenurses may experience the patient encounter by telephone as a conflict between being a carer and being a gatekeeper. An additional conflict for the telenurses may be knowing what is best for the patient and knowing the limited resources of health care.[11] Telenurses also feel considerable responsibility and have a fear of making the wrong decision.[10]

Calls with only some information exchange such as opening hour at a clinic are about 10% of calls to SHD (Ferm I., 2009, Personal Communication). About 50% of Swedish calls result in self-care advice only.[25] Furthermore, about 85% of callers are satisfied with the SHD services and about 92% report that they follow the advice they receive from telenurses (Ferm I., 2009, Personal Communication). In total, about 80% of the Swedish population know about SHD, the telephone number 1177, (Ferm I., 2009, Personal Communication) and its status as "care level zero."

In an effort to enhance medical safety within telenursing, books and CDSS are used[15] and medical safety and efficiency are considered main priorities.[23] Telenurses working at SHD use a CDSS intended to support their assessment and detect serious conditions. The Swedish CDSS used by the telenurses at SHD is one part of the telephone network.[20] The CDSS covers various symptoms and conditions common among children, adolescences, adults, and older people. It is symptom based on approximate 121 headings corresponding to common reasons for seeking advice. It suggests key questions based on the callers' symptoms (e.g., cough). Based on the callers' responses the CDSS suggests a recommended measure. Possible outcomes of a call include self-care advice, an appointment with a GP, a visit to the accident and emergency department, or request for an ambulance.[16] The CDSS can also be searched for specific information by entering a tentative diagnosis (e.g., migraine) and facts and recommendations are posed by the CDSS.[19] When choosing a symptom in the CDSS, the software forces the telenurses to follow it through.[1] If a Swedish telenurse overrides the recommendations in the CDSS, she then has to make a deviation report, stating why she chose to make a different recommendation.[1] When the texts with medical content are written, before inclusion in the CDSS, they are checked first by nurses, and then by physicians and other experts. Eventually the text will be approved by a board consisting of GPs before printing (Fig. 12.1).

The telenurses have described both pros and cons with CDSS.[7,9] The positive aspects are the use of CDSS for assessment and a feeling of having a safety net to rely on and provider of consistency. The negative aspects of the CDSS are that the software was experienced as not fully adapted to local practice and the program lacked in update, particularly the self-care advice was in need of update.

12.2.2
Policy and Operational Challenges

Callers have to pass the telenurses to get entrance to health care, and in that perspective the telenurses have considerable power. However, callers sometimes look upon telenurses as secretaries, who should not assess needs of care but give doctor's appointments according to the patients' wishes.[14] Another issue for Swedish telenurses to deal with is the problem of collaboration in the health-care sector. Wahlberg et al.[27] stated that it was difficult for telenurses to get district nurses or physicians to take over responsibility for the caller. Ernesäter et al.[6] have analyzed incident reports of errors related to Swedish telenursing and how these are handled. It seems from that study that it is easy to create a vicious circle where callers are referred around in the system, which is not only annoying, but also a threat to patient safety. For example, a caller talks to a telenurse at SHD who assesses the caller's symptoms. She decides, after recommendations from the CDSS that the caller needs to have a GP appointment within 24 h. Hence, the caller has to make a new call to his/her GP's surgery. Often the caller starts this second call by saying that the telenurse at SHD told him/her to get a GP appointment. However, this second nurse does not see it as

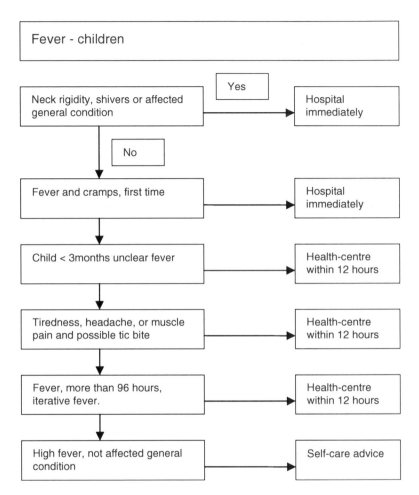

Fig. 12.1 Example of computerized decision support for the telenurse triage in fever children. The text is symptom based, with headings that correspond to common symptoms. Every title consists of a main symptom with a number of subsymptoms. The symptom boxes help the telenurse pose relevant questions to exclude or confirm serious conditions. For each symptom, there is a recommended level of urgency

her task to act on the telenurse's order. Instead, she starts a new assessment which might end up with a different recommendation, which in turn might make the caller uncertain, angry or scared, or a combination of these. This vicious circle is counterproductive for telenursing, the health-care sector, and society as a whole, and exactly what telenursing services were created to avoid. If the emergency department is too high a care level for the caller's symptoms, the care is not cost efficient and might take time from patients in more acute need of care. This is identified as a risk factor and a pattern that needs to be broken. However, as pointed out by Tjora,[22] callers' behavior is difficult to predict and they might choose to attend the emergency department despite having been given proper self-care advice. Even though callers rely on telenurses for medically safe advice, telenurses at the same time hand over considerable responsibility to the caller and rely on the caller's own ability to make sound judgments. In the quote below a telenurse describes a situation, which might have had a fatal ending.[11]

> This mother seemed like a normal mum to me... I thought that I'd thoroughly explained to her how to proceed. I told her that the baby had to see a doctor today... something made me call her again before I left my shift. And she was very happy for my call, and I heard from her description that her baby was in a much worse condition. She had called to the local GP but they had no acute appointments left – and then she just did nothing....

According to The National Board of Health and Welfare (1993), all registered nurses are obliged to make patient records when giving advice to callers. Furthermore, Swedish telenurses are personally liable for the caller. Hence, the telenurses, not the organization, take on the professional responsibility for their assessment and actions taken. At worst, the telenurse's registration or license might be withdrawn if the telenurse fails in some way. The telenurses have described that they almost always have this threat in the back of their minds while working. On the other hand, they are painstakingly aware that in their gate-keeping function, they cannot give every caller a doctor's appointment just to feel secure.[10] However, they are generous about giving doctors' appointment to small children and non-native Swedish speakers because their symptoms are harder to assess.

The Nordic countries have organized telecare in different ways. This is interesting to note since the Nordic countries have many other factors in common such as large rural areas (except Denmark), a similar infrastructure, common health problems, and rather similar political agendas. None of Sweden's neighboring countries has developed a telenursing call center organization in exactly the same way as in Sweden. However, while Finland and Norway have organized telecare in quite similar manners as Sweden, with telenurses giving advice to callers, Denmark has chosen a different organization. In Denmark, most patients are likely to call their own GP for advice when ill, at least during daytime. In 1992, a reform was launched in Denmark aiming to transfer both costs and working hours from out-of-hour periods to daytime. After this reorganization of out-of-hour work, callers have direct telephone access to a GP during out-of-hours. The GP on call has a triaging function, and assesses and decides whether the caller needs to be seen by a doctor, either at the surgery or at his/her home, or if the symptoms can be handled over the phone. It is emphasized that only experienced GPs should handle the telephone triage and advice.[4] Recently, however, it seems as Denmark will also start out telenursing services in line with other Western countries.

12.3
Future Direction

12.3.1
Program Expansion

Telenursing has been criticized for not being "real nursing,"[18] which might delay the process of developing a specialist university training course for telenurses. A formal telenursing education could build on three cornerstones: (1) medicine and nursing; (2) IT, telephone equipment, and other technology; and (3) communication. Quite some effort has been put into the development of the communication process in SHD. Nurses working at the SHD are educated to use a specific process ("Samtalsprocessen"). It contains five distinct phases: opening, listening, analyzing, motivating, and ending. Unfortunately, this communication process is not underpinned by scientific evidence although it has much in common with other models for communication.

Currently in Sweden short university courses in telenursing are provided by some universities and university colleges. These courses give 7.5–15 ECTS. The aims of these short courses differ between universities. For instance, the focus might be on the medical aspects, such as symptoms, diseases, and treatment in a rather traditional way to increase nurses' medical knowledge and provide opportunities for high medical safety. Other courses provide more of an overview of telenursing, and there are some courses with communication and dialogue between caller and telenurses as the core subject. A university course has also been given based on a CDSS. Several non-university courses are provided by different agencies and companies, 1–4 days in length. These courses can be rather expensive, whereas university courses are free of charge in Sweden.

In my personal experience, telenurses often ask for more education in three specific areas: (1) how to use their voice in a way that will ease the communication and allow them to talk constantly during a whole working day without getting a sore throat, (2) how to handle assertive or aggressive callers to avoid or solve conflicts, and (3) how to handle cross-cultural encounters where problems occur not only related to language issues, but also based on differing views on illness and health, the health-care system, and the role of telenurses. All three areas are part of communication aspects.

12.3.2
Policy and Goals of Telenursing

The communication process is an important area for further clinical development and research. Furthermore, I think that telenurses' educational role in relation to callers has to be strengthened. Because many calls, in some studies as much as 50%, result in self-care advice only, the educational strategies of telenurses used should be of importance. Telenurses have the opportunities of solving not only here and now problems, but also to empower and educate the callers, that is, the public, in health matters and self-care.[13] Potentially, if they can increase the self-care ability among only a small percentage of callers, public health might improve considerably.

However, this goal might not be achieved if telenurses, managers, and politicians do not see education and empowerment as part of the telenursing role. Hitherto, it seems that the educational role of telenursing work has not been emphasized by employers. This would certainly be an appropriate perspective for the authorities. Besides the general responsibility for a healthy population and health-promoting work according to the Swedish health-care act concerning all health and medical care, there is also a responsibility, when suitable, to inform about methods to prevent illness and harm (www.fhi.se). Moreover, the ICN code of ethics for nurses speaks about promoting health, preventing illness, and restoring health as three of four fundamental responsibilities (the last one is alleviating suffering) (www.icn.ch/icncode.pdf). This ethical code of nursing of course applies also in (Swedish) telenursing.

While in recent years efforts have been made to make telenursing accessible, medically safe and efficient, the time might now have come to develop the professional role of telenurses further and improve their educational competence. In a recent Swedish interview study of telenurses, only a few nurses described a comprehensive view of their task including to work with callers' understandings of symptoms and treatment.[13] Furthermore, a need for increased competence building regarding ethics[11] and gender-related aspects[8] has been identified within Swedish telenursing.

Call center-organized telenursing is likely to continue to expand in Sweden. In addition, technical solutions to assure medical safety and provide telenurses with more information on which to base their assessments will continue to develop. It is important that telenurses engage in such a development as active partners, otherwise we might risk getting solutions, which IT technicians and administrators find suitable, but which are not fully adapted for telenursing practice. However, promising technical solutions are already at hand in other parts of the world, where, for example, webcams and photos are used as complementary aids for telenursing assessment. In the near future also Swedish telenurses will surely have the possibility of checking, for instance, eczemas online while they talk to the caller. Online care and advice is already provided, but currently in a rather small-scale manner. This will probably be a more common task for telenurses in general within a few years. Might we then call the profession IT-mediated nursing? Telenurses may also soon take on a responsibility for monitoring and the follow-up of patients who have been hospitalized or who have received treatment.

There is, however, a risk that technology will be a detriment to nurses' ability to take individual measures for callers. Telenurses have already described that they felt inhibited in their work by the use of CDSS and that it lowered their professional autonomy.[7] The software might cause the telenurses to spend less time on the callers because they spend so much time on searching in the system. Hence, technology could hinder telenurses from focusing their energy on the caller. This could lead to misunderstandings and misinterpretation of information given by the caller and perhaps to a decrease in safety. Technology can be perceived as a barrier between the nurse and the patient; moreover, personal relations are complicated when technology demands the telenurses' attention.[3] Hence, the telenurses' flexibility within their own work, decisions, and working environment is at stake when the linear and mechanistic worldview meets caring ideals. I would like to see a study where different telenursing sites working in different ways with decision aid support are compared regarding caller outcomes and also outcomes such as stress level and work satisfaction for nurses.

Moreover, I am concerned about the fact that Swedish telenurses must work under considerable time pressure. In a perfect world, each call should be allowed to take the time needed. I do not argue that very long calls are always more efficient and satisfactory than shorter calls. It is, however, noteworthy that assessing symptoms without visual cues is indeed a challenging and demanding task. Intense listening to the caller's descriptions and asking numerous questions to make a medically safe assessment takes time. It self-care advice is the preferred measure, communicating this and checking the caller's understanding of the advice demands even more time. Derkx et al.[5] have recently shown that within a Dutch context quality of communication was correlated to call length. When the symptoms are, for example, of psychiatric nature, it is reasonable to assume that such a call might need extra time. On the other hand, when a caller asks for merely some brief information, a short call is probably preferable. Again, education and competence in communication are crucial so that nurses will use the time they have optimally, not in a standardized way but one adjusted to each caller's need in a truly patient-centered way. (For a definition of patient centeredness, see, e.g., Mead and Bower[17]) Hence, I would also like to see formal university education for telenurses, as argued above.

Moreover, better collaboration between different services within health care is needed to provide safe and efficient care for the public. Today, the regional distribution of care and both private and public telenursing call centers creates a fragmented picture, which often is difficult for both the public and the professionals, to navigate in. As stated by a nurse in one of our studies[11]:

> Today…they [the callers] do not feel well and there is no one to turn to. No place to go. They are suffering, they are in the middle of a divorce or something. They haven't slept for nights. They are walking around like zombies, and yet they have to go to work. And they call every where to get an appointment, but they are always referred…. (Nurse 10)

In 2006, only about 56% of callers were content with the accessibility of health care over the phone.[21] This might mean that accessibility needs to be improved or that the public need to get a more realistic picture of what to expect. How should a caller know about which organization has the responsibility for what? When should a person call SHD if his/her child is sick? Alternatively, when should a person call the pediatric emergency department or maybe the GPs surgery? I think that this is an educational task to work with.

To summarize, telenursing in Sweden has great possibilities for development within a near future. To attract competent nurses and make them stay in this demanding but challenging profession, a good working environment, possibilities for continued workplace learning, as well as formal courses are needed.

12.4
Summary

- In Sweden, a national project for development of telenursing started in 1997. However, telenursing call centers emerged on a broad scale only by 2000–2001. The national telenursing helpline is SHD.
- Telenursing in Sweden has been shown to be cost-effective and time saving and to increase patient self-care ability. Furthermore, it provides an opportunity for health promotion.
- There is no one single education for telenurses in Sweden. However, there is a current discussion about the need for a formal telenursing university education, aimed at providing a solid practice for telenurses and, furthermore, to ensure that telenursing gets the same status as other nursing specialties.
- Telenursing services in Sweden are provided by registered nurses at SHD, at specialized departments such as pediatrics, pediatric clinics, and health-care centers, and also by the alarm number 112 for emergency issues.
- In an effort to enhance medical safety within telenursing, books, and CDSS are used and medical safety and efficiency are main priorities.

Acknowledgments I am indebted to the telenurses who willingly shared their experiences with us. A special thank to Sara Holmström for invaluable help with transcriptions and administrative work. Grants were received from The Swedish Research Council (Vetenskapsrådet), The Swedish Council for Social Research, and the Faculty of Medicine, Uppsala University.

Glossary

Cost-effective – Productive relative to the cost.

Patient centeredness – Patient centeredness could be defined as: partnership between practitioners and patient, so that patient can make decisions and participate in their own care.

References

1. Andersson Bäck M. Conceptions, conflicts and contradictions: in the introduction of a Swedish health call centre. Institutionen för arbetsvetenskap, University of Gothenburg, Gothenburg; 2008.
2. Arnetz B. Psychosocial challenges facing physicians of today. Soc Sci Med. 2001;52: 203-213.
3. Barnard A, Sandelowski M. Technology and human nursing care: (ir)reconcilable or invented difference? J Adv Nurs. 2001;34(3):367-375.
4. Bondo Christensen M, Olesen F. Out of hour's service in Denmark: evaluation five years after reform. BMJ. 1998;316:1502-1505.
5. Derkx H, Rethans J-JE, Maiburg BH, et al. Quality of communication during telephone triage at Dutch out-of-hours centres. Patient Educ Couns. 2009;74:174-178.
6. Ernesäter A, Engström M, Holmström I, Winblad U. Incident reporting in nurse-led national telephone triage in Sweden: the reported errors reveal a pattern that needs to be broken. J Telemed Telecare. 2010;16(5):243-247.
7. Ernesäter A, Holmström I, Engström M. Telenurses' experiences of working with computerized decision support: supporting, inhibiting and quality improving. J Adv Nurs. 2009;65(5): 1074-1083.
8. Höglund A, Holmström I. "It's easier to talk to a woman" – aspects of gender in Swedish telenursing. J Clin Nurs. 2008;17(22):2979-2986.
9. Holmström I. Decision aid software programs in telenursing: not used as intended? Experiences of Swedish telenurses. Nurs Health Sci. 2007;9(1):23-28.
10. Holmström I, Dall'Alba G. "Carer and gatekeeper" – conflicting demands in nurses' experiences of telephone advisory services. Scand J Caring Sci. 2002;16(2):142-148.
11. Holmström I, Höglund AT. The faceless encounter. Ethical dilemmas in telephone nursing. J Clin Nurs. 2007;16(10):1865-1871.
12. Ipsos-Eureka. Vårdråd per telefon. Utvärdering av sjukvårdsrådgivningen i fyra landsting [Health care direct. Evaluation of the Swedish Health Direct in four counties]. Landstingsförbundet, Vårdråd per telefon, Stockholm; 2004.
13. Kaminsky E, Rosenqvist U, Holmström I. Telenurses' understanding of work: detective or educator? J Adv Nurs. 2009;65(2):382-390.

14. Leppänen V. *Telefonsamtal till Primärvården: Problem – Utforskning – Åtgärd (Telephone Calls to Primary Health Care: Problems – Investigation – Measures)*. Lund: Studentlitteratur; 2002.

15. Marklund B. Symtom, Råd, Åtgärd. Vårdutveckling AB, Vänersborg; 2000.

16. Marklund B, Ström M, Månsson J, et al. Computer-supported telephone nurse triage: an evaluation of medical quality and costs. *J Nurs Manag*. 2007;15(2):180-187.

17. Mead N, Bower P. Patient-centred consultations and outcomes in primary care: a review of the literature. *Patient Educ Couns*. 2002;48:51-61.

18. Snooks H, Williams AM, Griffith LJ, et al. Real nursing? The development of telenursing. *J Adv Nurs*. 2008;61:631-640.

19. Strom M, Marklund B, Hilding C. Nurses' perceptions of providing advice via a telephone care line. *Br J Nurs*. 2006;15(20):1119-1124.

20. Swedin B. Vårdråd direkt: sjukvårdsrådgivningar i samverkan: slutrapport från utredningen om nationellt samordnad sjukvårdsrådgivning. Landstingsförbundet, Stockholm; 2003.

21. Sveriges Kommuner och Landsting. Vårdbarometern: befolkningens syn på vården 2006 report. (The publics' views on health care during 2006). Sveriges kommuner och landsting, Stockholm; 2007.

22. Tjora A. Calls for Care: *Coordination, Competence, and Computers in Medical Emergency Call Centres*. Saarbrücken: Verlag Dr. Müller; 2009.

23. Valsecchi R, Andersson M, Smith C, et al. Tele-nursing: the English and Swedish experiences. In: 25th Annual Labour Process Conference; 2007; AIAS, Amsterdam.

24. Wahlberg A. Telephone advice nursing. Callers' perceptions, nurses experience of problems and basis for assessments. Department of Nursing, Karolinska Institute, Stockholm; 2004.

25. Wahlberg A, Wredling R. Telephone nursing: calls and caller satisfaction. *Int J Nurs Pract*. 1999;5:164-170.

26. Wahlberg AC, Cedersund E, Wredling R. Factors and circumstances related to complaints in emergency medical dispatching in Sweden: an exploratory study. *Eur J Emerg Med*. 2003;10(4):272-278.

27. Wahlberg A, Cedersund E, Wredling R. Telephone nurses' experience of problems with telephone advice in Sweden. *J Clin Nurs*. 2003;12(1):37-45.

Telenursing in the UK: A Brief Profile of National Health Service Direct

13

Julie Peconi, Helen Snooks, and Alison Porter

Abbreviations

CCDS	Computerized clinical decision support
GP	General practitioner
NHS	National Health Service
NHS 24	National Health Service 24
NHSD	National Health Service Direct
NHSDW	National Health Service Direct Wales
UK	United Kingdom

13.1
Introduction

The responsibility for health and well-being in the United Kingdom (UK) falls to the National Health Service (NHS). The NHS was established in 1948 to promote "the establishment of a comprehensive health service designed to secure improvement in the physical and mental health of the people of England and Wales and the prevention, diagnosis and treatment of illness" (NHS Act, 1946). The service varies from health-care provision in other Western countries, in that responsibility falls to the government in power.[37] As a result of changes in political administration and alongside changes in health, an aging population and advances in technology, over the past 60 years the NHS has experienced many adaptations, not only in the manner of delivery of health-care services, but also in the structure and organization of these services.

The NHS has recently undergone a series of changes in an attempt to bring the service up to date with economic, technological, medical, and social conditions. The explicit aim

J. Peconi (✉)
Centre for Health Information, Research and Evaluation (CHIRAL), College of Medicine, Swansea University, Singleton Park, Swansea, SA2 8PP, UK
e-mail: j.peconi@swansea.ac.uk

S. Kumar and H. Snooks (eds.), *Telenursing*, Health Informatics,
DOI: 10.1007/978-0-85729-529-3_13, © Springer-Verlag London Limited 2011

is to modernize the NHS to meet public expectations.[8] This includes an increased emphasis on the provision of care in the community, self-care, and prevention, with a parallel shift in the role of the general practitioner (GP). In the emergency care context, modernization is also taking place with the 2001 Reforming Emergency Care policy document complimenting the wider NHS modernization agenda.[27]

One important element of modernization which makes full use of technological advances in communication is telenursing, the provision of nursing services through means other than face-to-face contact. This chapter focuses on one aspect of telenursing in the UK, through the medium of 24-h nurse-led telephone helplines: NHS Direct (NHSD) in England, NHS Direct Wales (NHSDW), and NHS 24 in Scotland. The services provide health information and advice, often in emergency situations, and signpost callers to onward services if needed, for the cost of a local phone call. The aim of this chapter is to provide a brief history of these services, a picture of current use, and the role of nursing in NHSD, while highlighting issues of access and implications for the future.

13.2
Introducing NHSD, NHSDW, and NHS 24

In September 1997, the Chief Medical Officer for England's "Developing Emergency Services in the Community" recommended improving access to the NHS by the provision of emergency help and advice through a telephone helpline.[2] Shortly afterward, the British Government published a white paper, "The New NHS: Modern, Dependable", in which a 24-h nurse-led telephone health-care advice and information line – NHSD – was introduced in England. The service was followed quickly by similar services in Wales and Scotland. The aim of NHSD was to provide "easier and faster advice and information to people about health, illness, and the NHS, so that they are better able to care for themselves and their families."[7] The service was to empower patients while acting as a 24-h signpost to the multilayered NHS, directing callers to the most appropriate level of care. The specific objectives for the new service, set out by the Department of Health, the government department responsible for public health issues, included[23]:

- To offer the public a confidential, reliable, and consistent source of professional advice on health care, 24 h a day, so that they can manage many of their problems at home or know where to turn to for appropriate care.
- To provide simple and speedy access to a comprehensive and up-to-date range of health and related information.
- To help improve quality, increase cost-effectiveness, and reduce unnecessary demands on other NHS services by providing a more appropriate response to the needs of the public.
- To allow professionals to develop their role in enabling patients to be partners in self-care, and help them to focus on those patients for whom their skills are most needed.

NHSD was launched in 1998 with three pilot sites. The service rapidly expanded, and the scheme became nationwide in November 2000, with 22 call centers established across the country. The service is believed to be the world's first national nurse telephone clinical assessment service.[38] In December 1999, NHSD Online was introduced, a website where information about clinical conditions and health-care guidance can be accessed free of charge.[37] Information kiosks and digital television have also been added.

In Wales, several policy documents[13,42] gave a commitment to await research findings from the pilot sites in England before implementing a national health helpline, although in practice comprehensive evidence about costs, impact and evidence was not produced before the service was expanded to cover both the whole of England and Wales.[16] In 1999, the Secretary of State announced the introduction of NHSDW. The service was to be commissioned by the Specialised Health Services Commission for Wales based in Swansea NHS Trust. It was operational in April 2000 in two areas, with the rest of Wales receiving service by December of the same year. The aims of NHSDW are similar to NHSD: "to help callers by providing the right advice, information and reassurance they require to look after themselves, if appropriate." It was also designed to ensure that callers who need further care are directed to the right service at the right time.[32]

In Scotland, the service is named NHS 24 and introduction followed a similar pattern. In March 1999, an initial announcement was made by the Secretary of State for the country that an investment was to be made in primary care to pilot the expansion of existing GP "out-of-hours" services to include 24-h access to nurse-led health advice. In December 2000, the service was officially named NHS 24 and was rolled out in pilot areas during 2001. However, while the new service in Scotland was to be similar to NHSD in England, in that nurse triage was to play a key role, there was a stronger focus on integration with existing services, including GP out-of-hours, ambulance, and pharmacists.[3]

Although these services are separately run in practice, in this chapter, for simplicity, the term "NHSD" is used to refer to all three (unless otherwise specified as relating to England), as they are so similar in objectives and organization.

13.3
How NHSD Works in Practice

At the time of writing, NHSD in England has 36 call centers across the country with over 3,000 employees – 1,200 of whom are nurses. All services operate similarly to call centers, in which employees work independently answering continuous calls from the public. There is an option for nurses to discuss calls with colleagues from other specialties although all calls are timed and recorded. As calls may be stressful, staff are given the opportunity to debrief following a shift.

13.3.1
The Call Handler

Although NHSD is referred to as a "nurse-led" service, calls to the service are first answered by a call handler who gathers basic information. The call handler will then direct the call to the most appropriate person – a nurse or health information advisor, depending on the nature of the query. If the condition of the caller or patient is not urgent, the call may then be put in a queue and the caller called back when the next appropriate person is available. By contrast, if the call handler deems the situation to be an emergency, he/she can call an ambulance immediately.

13.3.2
Health Information Referral

Health information advisors deal with enquiries about local services and requests for information about conditions, treatments, and procedures. In NHSD, approximately 13% of calls are handled by health information advisors who may or may not be medically qualified (many come from the social-care environment). Health information advisors also offer information on the prevention of ill health, such as referrals to local smoking cessation schemes. Information is supplied to the caller by phone, by post, or via the Internet.

13.3.3
The Nurse Advisor

NHSD nurse advisors come from a variety of backgrounds including midwifery, health visiting, pediatrics, accident and emergency, and community nursing. Nurse advisors do not make diagnoses but triage callers or patients, using computerized clinical decision support (CCDS) software called the Clinical Advice System. At the start of the telephone conversation, from the caller's responses to initial questions, the nurse decides which algorithm, or branch of the system, to follow, leading the caller through a series of questions resulting in advice concerning further health-care required, where to go for that care and when. This call outcome is termed the "disposition." At any stage in the conversation the nurse can override the system's recommended course of action but should document his/her reasons for doing so.

13.4
Research Evidence Concerning NHSD

Each of the three services (NHSD, NHSDW, and NHS 24) has undergone independent evaluations, with some consistent results across services.[3,22,23,41] Although these evaluations have shown that the services are generally well liked by the public, each also indicates that the speed of expansion has left many issues still to be explored. For example, in Scotland, an independent evaluation concluded the service's actual role had changed significantly compared with its intended role and many processes and procedures had not withstood the pressures of operation.[3] Key areas highlighted by the research evidence include the role of nursing in NHSD, call volume and patterns, impact on the demand for other services, clinical and cost-effectiveness, user satisfaction, and issues of access.

13.5
The Role of Nursing in NHSD

The introduction of NHSD was seen by some as a new career option for nurses and the service has provided employment for those with disabilities who otherwise may have had to leave the profession.[19] On the whole, NHSD nurses have been found to be generally satisfied with working for the service and have gained opportunities for skill development and promotion since joining, although a minority also have reported the work to be monotonous[14] and stressful.[40]

Although NHSD nurses use their professional clinical judgment to assess a caller's health and are only supported by the CCDS, there has been some debate about whether working in NHSD as a nurse advisor constitutes "real nursing," with nurses outside the service in particular expressing doubts.[40] This is understandable, given that telenursing differs from the traditional hands-on delivery of nursing care and there is still much work to be done to understand telephone-based clinical decision making and nursing practice issues. NHSD, as one of the "pioneers" for telephone-based delivery of public health care,[4] has been the setting for much of this research. Pettinari and Jessop[34] explored how professional knowledge and experience were used to build skills to manage the absence of visibility. They identified three broad areas in which nurses have adapted to manage the lack of copresence: (1) gathering information, (2) delivering information, and (3) building trust and rapport. In this way the nurse is able to build a picture of the client and his/her environment, a process seen as central to the reasoning process.[11] Despite this, stresses related to the lack of face-to-face contact with patients were found to be present with telephone nurse advisors both in NHSD in the UK[40] and in Sweden.[44]

Research has also focused on how nurses maintain their professional values within the restriction of the call center environment with its close monitoring. Evidence suggests that nurses use their professional clinical skills, as outcomes of assessments over the telephone by nurses vary,[29,30] indicating an interaction with the CCDS. Mueller et al. found that NHSD nurses display professionalism in four ways: safety of advice, negotiating conflicting expectations, monitoring and simulation, and the role of emotional labor and empathy. Overall, the researchers found evidence that in NHSD, empathy and caring are seen as a component of professional identify and are not due to managerial coercion.[20]

13.6
Service Use

The volume of calls to NHSD has increased steadily since its inception with almost five million calls taken in England on the direct number in 2007/2008.[26] Evaluations of NHSD and NHSDW found that the callers make contact with appropriate services following their call to NHSD in a large majority of cases. Furthermore, serious adverse events resulting from NHSD contract were likely to be rare.[22] However, evidence in Wales deemed the service to be expensive (average marginal cost per call £29 compared to £23 for a consultation with a GP).[41]

Callers appear to be extremely satisfied with their contacts with NHSD.[28] Of the callers who followed the advice given, 95% were satisfied[35] while in a separate study, 95% rated the advice and/or information given as excellent, very good, or good.[26] The website has also grown in popularity with almost 31 million hits in 2007/2008 (a tenfold increase over 5 years).[26]

Published results indicate that self-care advice accounts for the largest proportion of call outcomes,[26,33] with almost 50% of calls resulting in advice to self-care.[26] As one of the objectives of NHSD was to ease pressure on emergency and unscheduled care providers,[2] these data sound promising. However, although methodologically difficult to measure, evidence suggests that in its first year in England, NHSD did not reduce the demand for other immediate care service providers (accident and emergency, ambulance, and GP services) although it may have restrained increasing demand on GPs' out-of-hours services.[21] Using a similar methodology, no evidence of any substitution of demand for other service providers was found in Wales.[41]

13.7
Issues of Access

Equity of access has always been one of the fundamental aims of the NHS. Indeed, in the same white paper which announced the introduction of NHSD, fair access was cited as an important dimension of the new NHS framework: "The NHS contribution must begin by offering fair access to health services in relation to people's needs, irrespective of geography, class, ethnicity, age, or sex."[7] Despite this, concerns have been raised by evaluators,[12] policy makers,[25] and nurses[40] that NHSD is not reaching all of the population, with those who may be particularly vulnerable – older people, those living in areas of deprivation, and those from ethnic minority backgrounds – generally making much less use of the service than other groups such as young parents (who are particularly heavy users), the relatively well educated and affluent.

Published studies have looked at who uses NHSD by exploring access across many different patient groups. These studies looked at whether older people,[6] patients in general practice waiting rooms,[36,43] those from varying levels of deprivation,[1,5] and those who arrived at a hospital by ambulance[17] were aware of and had used the service. Two studies looked at a random sample of the general population[15,39] when attempting to explore access.

In two ecological studies (an investigation that involves a group, typically a geographically defined area, as the unit of analysis),[18] NHSD call rates rose with increasing deprivation but dropped off in the most deprived areas.[1,5] When figures were further broken down, Cooper et al.[5] found that the effect of extreme deprivation seemed to raise rates of calls about adults but reduce rates about children. At an individual level, results are similar, with questionnaires used to gather information on socioeconomic characteristics regarding the use of NHSD. Material deprivation significantly reduced the likelihood of using NHSD as well as non-UK birth of the head of the family.[39] Respondents were less likely to use NHSD if they were aged 65 or more, lacked access to a car or telephone, did not own their homes, had language or hearing difficulties, or had left full-time education at a young age.[15] There were conflicting results with respect to the relationship between use of the service and health status.[36,39]

Several studies compared levels of awareness of NHSD across different populations. Both David[6] and McInerney et al.[17] found that awareness of NHSD declined with age although there are mixed conclusions as to whether this lack of awareness impacted use by the elderly. David found that contacts with NHSD declined with age in line with levels of awareness, suggesting that older people were no less likely than younger ones to use the service if they were aware of it. In contrast, in a questionnaire survey of those in a general practice waiting room, Ullah et al.[43] found that even when aware of NHSD, older people were less like to use it with the most cited reasons for people over 50 not using it being that they preferred to see their GP.

Ambulatory patients from less affluent postcodes and those from ethnic minorities were also found to be less aware of the service,[17] although there were no differences in use or awareness of NHSD in ethnic group or social class.[43] It is, however, important to keep in mind that many of these studies took place shortly after the introduction of NHSD and levels of awareness today may have changed.

13.8
Discussion: Implications for Policy, Research, and Practice

In its first 10 years of existence, NHSD has grown in size, scope (expanding to include the website, digital television and information kiosks), and popularity with high levels of caller satisfaction. The service now handles calls to out-of-hours GP services in some parts of the country, as well as various other clinical assessment services, "choose and book" appointments. Work with local providers of urgent care is also underway to strengthen the integration of service provision.[10] Priorities for the future include building on the core service it provides and moving to a contract that would fit the new NHS environment, providing more enhanced services for customers; working more closely with other NHS organizations and integrated services, and being at the forefront to the application of new technologies to health care.[26]

Research evidence indicates that nurses are generally satisfied with working in NHSD and have adapted views on traditional "hands-on" nursing to fit the call center environment. However, it has been argued that NHSD has been introduced without a solid evidence base[16] and the speed of expansion has often made evaluation difficult, leaving many issues needing further exploration. In particular, the service has not been found to reduce the demand for other immediate care service providers and, in this way, has failed to meet one of its original intended objectives. Although it has been suggested that NHSD is offering an alternative route into the NHS for those concerned with being considered "time wasters" by other busy services,[31] the full reasons why this substitution of demand has not occurred are not yet understood.

In addition, levels of access from vulnerable groups (those who are economically deprived, of ethnic minority background or older than 65 years) are lower than the general population. These groups of the population are already disadvantaged in terms of their health status and access to services and are groups that could potentially stand to benefit the most from a confidential service within their own homes. Further research is needed to understand the reasons why these groups are not using the service fully and what can be done to improve equity of access.

Despite a lack of robust evidence concerning the achievement of NHSD's objectives, in practical terms the service is safe and well liked and would be politically difficult to decommission. Indeed, policy direction indicates that NHSD is to continue to form an integrated part of the health-care system.[9,24] However, in the resource-limited NHS environment, concerns about clinical and cost-effectiveness, and access by disadvantaged groups, need to be further explored in order to understand what value is added by the service, and how the service can be developed in such a way that its effectiveness and reach across the population are maximized.

13.9
Summary

- NHSD, NHSDW, and NHS 24 are 24-h nurse-led confidential health advice and information telephone services.
- The services' aims include the provision of "easier and faster advice and information to people about health, illness and the NHS, so that they are better able to care for themselves and their families."
- NHSD nurses are generally satisfied in working for the service and have adapted their role to fit the telenursing environment, although a small minority report the work to be monotonous and stressful.
- The services are well liked by the public with satisfaction rates as high as 95%.
- Advice to self-care accounts for the largest proportion of call outcomes, although the service has not shown to lessen the demand for other immediate care service providers.
- Despite call volumes increasing steadily, the service is underused by vulnerable groups (those who are economically deprived, of ethnic minority background or older than 65 years).
- NHSD continues to grow in size, scope, and popularity with policy direction indicating that it is to continue to form an integrated part of the UK health-care system.
- More research is needed to understand how the service can maximize its effectiveness and reach across the population.

Glossary

Computerized clinical decision support software – An electronic program that can aid in decision making and triage.

National Health Service – The organization responsible for health and well-being in the UK, which is the responsibility of the government in charge.

NHS Direct – A 24-h nurse-led confidential telephone helpline providing health-care advice and information to callers.

White paper – In the context of UK government policy, a white paper is a first draft of proposed legislation which will be subject to debate before becoming a law.

References

1. Burt J, Hooper R, Jessopp L. The relationship between use of NHS Direct and deprivation in southeast London: an ecological analysis. *J Public Health Med.* 2003;25(2):174-176.
2. Calman K. Developing emergency services in the community: the final report. NHS Executive, London; 1997.
3. Clarke O, Beacom B, Bell D, et al. Report: review of NHS 24. Independent review team; 2005.
4. Collin-Jacques C, Smith C. Nursing on the line: experiences from England and Quebec (Canada). *Hum Rel.* 2005;58(1):5-32.
5. Cooper D, Arnold E, Smith G, et al. The effect of deprivation, age and sex on NHS Direct call rates. *Br J Gen Pract.* 2005;55(513):287-291.
6. David OJ. NHS Direct and older people. *Age Ageing.* 2005;34(5):499-501.
7. Department of Health. The New NHS: Modern, Dependable. CMD, Editor. London: The Stationary Office; 1997.
8. Department of Health. The NHS Plan: A Plan for Investment, a Plan for Reform. HMSO, Editor. London; 2000.
9. Department of Health. *Reforming Emergency Care.* London: The Stationary Office; 2001.
10. Department of Health /Access Directorate – Primary Care Branch. NHS direct commissioning framework April 2006–March 2007; Guidance for Primary Care Trusts on Commissioning NHS Direct Services April 2006.
11. Edwards B. Seeing is believing – picture building: a key component of telephone triage. *J Clin Nurs.* 1998;7:51-57.
12. George S. NHS Direct audited. *BMJ.* 2002;324(7337):558-559.
13. Gregory P, Kennedy R. Welsh Health Circular: Management Arrangements for the Introduction and Operation of NHS Direct Wales. N. Division, Editor. The National Assembly for Wales; 1999.
14. Knowles E, O'Cathain A, Morrell J, et al. NHS Direct and nurses – opportunity or monotony? *Int J Nurs Stud.* 2002;39(8):857-866.
15. Knowles E, Munro J, O'Cathain A, et al. Equity of access to health care. Evidence from NHS Direct in the UK. *J Telemed Telecare.* 2006;12(5):262-265.
16. McDonnell A, Wilson R, Goodacre S. Evaluating and implementing new services. *BMJ.* 2006;332:109-112.
17. McInerney J, Chillala S, Read C, et al. Impact of NHS direct on demand for immediate care. Target communities show poor awareness of NHS Direct. *BMJ.* 2000;321(7268):1077.
18. Morgenstern H. Uses of ecologic analysis in epidemiologic research. *Am J Public Health.* 1982;72(12):1336-1344.
19. Morrell CJ, Munro J, O'Cathain A, et al. Impact of NHS Direct on other services: the characteristics and origins of its nurses. *Emerg Med J.* 2002;19(4):337-340.
20. Mueller F, Valsecchi R, Smith C, et al. 'We are nurses, we are supposed to care for people': professional values among nurses in NHS Direct call centres. *New Technol Work Employ.* 2008;23(1–2):2-16.
21. Munro J, Nicholl J, O'Cathain A, et al. Impact of NHS Direct on demand for immediate care: observational study. *BMJ.* 2000;321(7254):150-153.
22. Munro J, Nicholl J, O'Cathain A, et al. Evaluation of NHS Direct first wave sites: final report of the phase 1 research. MCR Unit, Editor. Sheffield University, Sheffield; 2001:102.

23. Munro J, Clancy M, Knowles E, et al. Evaluation of NHS Direct: impact and appropriateness. MCR Unit, Editor. Sheffield University, Sheffield; 2003.

24. National Assembly for Wales. *A Plan for the NHS with Its Partners: Improving Health in Wales*. Cardiff: National Assembly for Wales; 2001.

25. National Audit Office. NHS Direct in England. T.S. Office, Editor. National Audit Office, London; 2002.

26. NHS Direct. Annual Report & Accounts. A year of success. T.S. Office, Editor. London; 2007/2008.

27. Nicholl J. Reforming emergency care. *Emerg Med J.* November 2001;3-4.

28. O'Cathain A, Munro JF, Nicholl JP, et al. How helpful is NHS Direct? Postal survey of callers. *BMJ.* 2000;320(7241):1035.

29. O'Cathain A, Webber E, Nicholl J, et al. NHS Direct: consistency of triage outcomes. *Emerg Med J.* 2003;20(3):289-292.

30. O'Cathain A, Nicholl J, Sampson F, et al. Do different types of nurses give different triage decisions in NHS Direct? A mixed methods study. *J Health Serv Res Policy.* 2004;9(4):226-233.

31. O'Cathain A, Goode J, Luff D, et al. Does NHS Direct empower patients? *Soc Sci Med.* 2005;61(8):1761-1771.

32. Parker M. Welsh health circular: NHS Direct Wales and primary care – liability issues. N. Division, Editor. The National Assembly for Wales; 2001.

33. Payne F, Jessopp L. NHS Direct: review of activity data for the first year of operation at one site. *J Public Health Med.* 2001;23(2):155-158.

34. Pettinari CJ, Jessopp L. "Your ears become your eyes": managing the absence of visibility in NHS Direct. *J Adv Nurs.* 2001;36(5):668-675.

35. IFF Research Ltd. NHS Direct appropriateness and timeliness of referrals; 2008. Research Report prepared for NHS Direct.

36. Ring F, Jones M. NHS Direct usage in a GP population of children under 5 years: is NHS Direct used by people with the greatest health need? *Br J Gen Pract.* 2004;54(500):211-213.

37. Rivett GC. *Cradle to Grave: Fifty Years of the NHS*. London: King's Fund; 1998.

38. Sadler M, Challiner J. Calls to NHS Direct. *Emerg Med J.* 2008;25(1):59.

39. Shah SM, Cook DG. Socio-economic determinants of casualty and NHS Direct use. *J Public Health (Oxf).* 2008;30(1):75-81.

40. Snooks H, Williams A, Griffiths L, et al. Real nursing? The development of telenursing. *J Adv Nurs.* 2001;61(6):631-640.

41. Snooks H, Behi R, Cheung WY, et al. NHS Direct Wales evaluation final report February 2006. Swansea University, Swansea; 2006.

42. Williams RC, Hall D, Bull MP. NHS Direct Wales. T. Chief Executives – Health Authorities, Directors of Public Health, Directors of Patient Care, Directors of Contractor Services, General Practitioners, LMC's, GMSC (Wales), PSNC (Wales), WMC, WNMC, Editor. Welsh Office, Cardiff, p. Letter; 1998.

43. Ullah W, Theivendra A, Sood V, et al. Men and older people are less likely to use NHS Direct. *BMJ.* 2003;326(7391):710.

44. Wahlberg A, Cedersund E, Wredling R. Telephone nurses' experience of problems with telephone advice in Sweden. *J Clin Nurs.* 2003;12:37-45.

Supporting the UK Patient with a Long-Term Condition: Policy, Strategy, Education, and Telehealth

14

Susan Bell and Ann Saxon

Abbreviations

COPD	Chronic Obstructive Pulmonary Disease
ICT	Information and Communication Technology
IT	Information Technology
KSF	Knowledge and Skills Framework
NHS	National Health Service
NPfIT	National Programme for Information Technology
SCT	Scottish Center for Telehealth
TSA	Telecare Services Association
UK	United Kingdom
WAG	Welsh Assembly Government

14.1
The Need for Change

The sheer number of people with a long-term condition requiring care in the community continues to grow, but the number of health professionals available to provide the care is declining. Even with a current National Health Service (NHS) workforce of around 1.3 million, a number exceeded only by the Chinese Army and the shopping chain Wal-Mart, the NHS is struggling to meet the current demand on resources, let alone the demands of the future. The financial cost to the NHS in 2008 was approaching £2 billion/week.[8]

With increasing pressure on resources throughout the health service in the UK a significant change is needed in the way services are provided and care is delivered.

S. Bell (✉)
Choose Independence, Peterborough, UK
e-mail: susieboo13@hotmail.com

S. Kumar and H. Snooks (eds.), *Telenursing*, Health Informatics,
DOI: 10.1007/978-0-85729-529-3_14, © Springer-Verlag London Limited 2011

14.2
Changes in the Provision of Health and Social Care in the UK

It is now over 10 years since the constitutional devolution of governance for health care to the separate UK countries, England, Wales, Scotland, and Ireland. Each country has developed plans to meet future health and social care needs, and a brief overview of the strategy of each country is given.

All four countries have a national program for information and communication technology. While progress in each country is at different stages of implementation, the common aim of each country is the development of a single electronic patient record.

In Wales the program is called Informing Health Care (www.wales.nhs.uk/ihc), in Scotland the e-Health program (www.ehealthscot.nhs.uk).

In Northern Ireland the program is called the HPSS ICT Programme (www.dhsspsni.gov. uk) and in England it is called Connecting for Health (www.connectingforhealth.nhs.uk).

For more information about the development and quality of care in the four devolved countries, the reader is directed to "Quality in Healthcare in England, Wales, Scotland, Northern Ireland: an intra UK Chart book," produced by The Health Foundation.[16]

Alternatively, the NHS websites of the individual countries, www.nhs.england, www. nhs.wales, www.nhsscotland, and www.nhsireland contain useful information.

14.2.1
Wales

In May 2005, the Welsh Assembly Government (WAG) published "Designed for Life – Creating World Class Health and Social Care for Wales in the 21st Century," a strategy for health and social care in Wales.[19] The 10-year strategy is underpinned by three aims: life-long health, fast safe and effective services, and world-class care which will be achieved through good partnerships between the NHS, public health, local government, and voluntary organizations, working toward a single goal of improving the quality of life in Wales.

14.2.2
Scotland

The white paper "Partnership for Care"[17] (www.scotland.gov.uk/publications) sets out a clear direction for NHS Scotland, decentralizing power and involving patients, staff, and the public in improving services. Measures recommended include redesign of services and better integration and partnership, so that the patient experiences a quicker service. The consultation document "Better Health Better Care"[18] recognizes the potential offered by all aspects of telehealth as a way forward in improving health care in Scotland.

The Scottish Centre for Telehealth (SCT), an advisory body, shares information on successes in telehealth across the world. The SCT "would encourage the establishment of a large scale project in 'telehomecare' in the management of long-term conditions" (www. scottish.parliament.uk/s3).

14.2.3
Northern Ireland

In 2002, The Review of Public Administration was launched to deliver wide ranging modernization and reform of health, education, and local government. The newly formed Health and Social Care Board for Northern Ireland will focus on commissioning, resource management, performance management, and improvement. The newly formed Patient and Client Council will replace the current Health and Social Services Council to represent the voice of patients, clients, and carers (www.northernireland.gov.uk).

Northern Ireland will develop a new European Centre for Connected Health to bring telehealth solutions to 5,000 people by 2011 and aim to reduce the number of hospital admissions by 50% by 2011. The initiative will concentrate on three chronic conditions, chronic obstructive pulmonary disease (COPD), chronic heart failure, and diabetes.

14.2.4
England

Professor the Lord Darzi of Denham identified recommendations for change in "High Quality Care for All."[8] The report outlines the "vision of an NHS that gives patients and the public more information and choice, works in partnership, and has quality of care at its heart – quality defined as clinically effective, personal and safe," and clearly sets out the changes to be made to achieve this vision.

The report states that systems must be speeded up to improve access to health services, and a significant reduction in the time a patient waits to begin treatment or receive care or services as needed.

Lord Darzi also maintains that health care must continue to be free for all users. Free care for all has been the mantra of the NHS since its beginnings in the mid-1940s, although in some areas of the UK patients now pay for their medicines.

Another recommendation of Lord Darzi is the introduction of a new NHS constitution[10] with the involvement of the public, patients, and staff contributing to the content. The constitution "establishes the principles and values in England by which all NHS bodies and private and third sector providers supplying NHS services will be required by law to take account of in their decisions and actions.". The purpose is to ensure providers meet the expectations of the public, patients, and staff through the provision of high-quality care.

14.3
Tomorrow's Workforce

Changes are needed to modify the careers of nurses, doctors, dentists, and allied health professionals. The review "A High Quality Workforce"[7] outlines the roles of tomorrow's nurses, doctors, dentists, and allied health professionals, and proposes that changes in these roles are needed to develop the "right workforce to provide safe, high quality patient services in the future." The review discusses the need for clear educational pathways to equip professionals with the knowledge they need to perform their individual role well.

Sources of further information about modernizing nurses' and allied health professionals' careers are The Modernising Nursing Careers Programme[6] (www.dh.gov.uk/en/Publications) and the Modernising Allied Health Professions Careers Project[9] (www.dh.gov.uk/en/publications).

Clarity is essential in determining the knowledge and skills health professionals need. The Knowledge and Skills Framework (KSF) is in simple terms a set of performance indicators associated with each job and is also linked to educational and training needs. The KSF was introduced under "Agenda for Change" in 2004.[13]

Agenda for Change is the biggest overhaul of NHS-wide pay, terms and conditions in 50 years (www.rcn.org.uk/agendaforchange).

Another useful source which describes competencies health care professionals require is (www.skillsforhealth.org.uk). The competencies describe what individuals need to do, what they need to know and which skills they need to carry out an activity. Skills for Health competencies can be used by all levels of health staff in the NHS, independent and voluntary sector. The aim of competency-based practice is to ensure that activities carried out every day by health-care workers across the UK are performed effectively and consistently.

14.4
The Community Matron: A New Nursing Role in England

The NHS Improvement Plan[3] describes a new clinical role for nurses, that of the community matron, who would "use case management techniques with patients who meet a criteria denoting very high intensity use of health care resources" and that "with special intensive help these patients will be able to remain living at home longer and have more choice about their health care." The principle of this model of case management is that there is one person who acts both as provider and procurer of care who "takes responsibility for ensuring all health and social care needs are met."

Case management aims to prevent unnecessary hospital admissions and reduce the length of stay associated with necessary hospital admissions. Discharge planning ensures that the support a patient will need on return home is in place before discharge. Crosbie[1] describes the discharge planning as process as "a collective activity with multidisciplinary contribution being key to success." The principle of "early referral to community nursing services, social services, physiotherapy or occupational services promotes consideration of the patient's medical, personal, functional and social circumstances" highlighting the need for careful forward planning.

"Achieving timely simple discharge from hospital: A toolkit for the multidisciplinary team" published in 2004[2] helps staff to identify, plan, and arrange care or support the patient will need. Communication between the nurse planning discharge and the community matron therefore is essential to ensure continuity of care.

A highly skilled practitioner, the community matron, is able to deliver evidence-based practice in accordance with the most up-to-date guidelines and recommendations, co-ordinate care or services from all other agencies and prescribe medicines. Their knowledge, expertise, and extensive skills take time to develop and are underpinned with academic achievement. The Skills for Health competencies have proved to be valuable in shaping the proactive aspect of the community matron role (www.skillsforhealth.org.uk).

14.4.1
Community Matrons and Long-Term Conditions Developing Essential Skills

It is estimated that 17.5 million people are living with a long-term condition in the UK[5] and several of those people require hospitalization for their condition. In 2005 the role of the community matron/case manager was introduced in the UK[4] to support patients with long-term conditions and help support them in their own homes and prevent unnecessary hospital admissions. The World Health Organisation[20] have predicted that chronic health conditions will be a leading cause of disability by the year 2020 and if not managed in an appropriate way will become an expensive problem for all nations. Many people in the UK have complex health needs which need to have specialist support and guidance.

The majority of people who have a long-term condition have complex health needs and require the skills of specialist practitioners to support them, in particular in the home setting. The role of the community matron has developed mainly from the work in the United States and the work of Evercare[11] and Kaiser Permanente (www.kaiserpermanente.org). The role encompasses that of care navigator and care provider ensuring that people have the right services at the right time to support them.

The Department of Health[5] identified a range of skills that are required to support patients with chronic long-term conditions. Skills for Health[4] published the case management competencies framework, which was underpinned by the principles laid out in the NHS health and social care model for people with long-term conditions.[5]

The competencies would enable the development of a range of skills as a community matron or case manager. They define the roles and responsibilities as follows:

The community matron will provide a full case management service, typically for a caseload of 50 very-high-intensity users. They will provide clinical nursing in the home.

The case manager will usually be a qualified nurse, social worker, or allied health professional. They will work with individuals who have a dominant complex single condition, for example, diabetes or chest conditions without complications.[5]

The following have been identified as some of the essential skills of this role:

- Advanced assessment skills
- Advanced clinical skills
- Case management
- Role development
- Collaborative working
- Case management

Advanced assessment skills: People with long-term conditions have a plethora of symptoms of their condition which can affect their ability to function on a day-to-day basis. The community matron is required to utilize a range of advanced skills that ordinarily would not be required of practitioners in this care setting. The use of an assessment framework is recommended to ensure that all of the key issues have been identified and planned for in a package of care.

Essential skills include the following:

- Verbal and non-verbal communication skills
- Listening skills
- History taking
- Holistic assessment skills
- Care planning
- Care evaluation

The advanced clinical nursing skills are identified as:

- Advanced clinical assessment skills
- Risk assessment and appropriate management of risk
- Advanced ability to use information to undertake assessments, including clinical decision making and judgment
- In-depth knowledge of the pathophysiology of conditions, and the presentation and prognosis of long-term conditions
- In-depth knowledge of therapeutic interventions including pharmacology and medicines management
- In-depth knowledge of the current legislation and the ethical principles which underpin care of this dimension
- Sophisticated application of holistic person-centered models of care

Advanced nurses working in this role will have highly developed and have usually undertaken studies at master's level. They will have detailed skills in taking a comprehensive patient history and carrying out a physical examination of their patients with a long-term condition. They will use their expert knowledge and judgment to identify the potential diagnosis and refer patients for investigations where appropriate. They will be able to make a final diagnosis and use their expert skills to develop and provide skilled competent care. Community matrons can access patient records, review test results, and make referrals to local services at the touch of a button, reducing waiting time to access services and start treatment.

Nurses working in this role will also have completed extra training and education in the prescribing and management of medicines in the community setting, enabling them to provide a whole service from diagnosis of the current problem, through to a program of treatment and evaluation of care.

14.4.2
Quality of Life

For many patients with a chronic condition it is not only the physical problems they have to encounter on a day-to-day basis, but the emotional strain can lead to problems such as anxiety and depression.[12]

The community matron will have developed skills in identifying those patients who need some psychological support and provide referral for treatment of anxiety and depression. For example, they may be involved in the following areas:

- The use of assessment tools in mental health care
- Appropriate referral to counseling services and psychological support therapies
- Recognizing the signs of depression
- Self-management tools that patients can access
- Referral to specialist mental health practitioners
- Advanced communication skills

The community matron will use the above skills to coordinate services to patients with psychological needs and identify those most at risk.

In addition to the range of advanced skills the community matron can provide it is also import patients with a long-term condition are encouraged and supported to manage the conditions themselves where possible. The aim of encouraging self help is to encourage active involvement in their care, the community matron will also develop a range of skills in promoting health and preventing ill health, which help the patient to stay as well as they can within the confines of their condition.

These skills will include the following:

- Skills in analyzing, interpreting, and presenting public health data
- Knowledge and understanding of evaluation methods and the ethical principles associated with this
- In-depth knowledge of the social constructs of health and illness
- Self-help skills, in particular motivational interviewing

The education and training of this group of practitioners has been developed since 2005 and a variety of methods of education have been established, from more formal courses to the use of e-technology in blended and e-learning programs. There is a constant need for all practitioners to remain confident and competent in their area of practice to ensure that patients with a long-term condition remain supported.

14.5
Improving Care and Services Through Technology

While new strategies, policies, and role redesign underpin the changes in the way health and social care will be provided, a smarter way of working is needed too. With the explosion of innovative technology, this is not just a possibility, but a reality. Technology is playing a key role in the development of the NHS of the future.

The NHS is under pressure to "speed things" up. The National Programme for Information Technology in the NHS (referred to as the program or NPfIT) was set up to provide high-quality services to patients in England (www.publications.parliament.uk). Central to NPfIT is the NHS Care Records Service, set up to replace local NHS computer systems with more modern integrated systems and make key elements of a patient's clinical record available throughout England.

The electronic "summary care record" (www.nhscarerecords/nhs/uk) contains information about the patient, and can be accessed and contributed to by all health professionals involved in the patient's care. At present, there is a heated debate about the sheer volume of information the record will contain and how quickly specific information can be accessed by a health-care professional, but the attraction of quick access and paperless record keeping is at the heart of this initiative.

NPfIT also includes the introduction of electronic prescriptions, NHS e-mail which is a 99.5% secure system, a directory service of all NHS staff (NHS mail), computer-accessible X-rays (picture archive communication systems) and a facility for patients to electronically book first outpatient appointments with a specialist.

Choose and book (www.chooseandbook.nhs.uk) enables a patient to choose an appointment at a date and time convenient for them, cutting out the waiting time between referral and appointment.

A clinical dashboard is a toolset developed to provide clinicians with timely and relevant information, giving clinicians easy access to the wealth of NHS data whenever they need it.

The Clinical Dashboards Programme (www.connectingforhealth.nhs.uk/systemsandservices/clindash/overview) has been established within the previously mentioned English information technology (IT) program, Connecting for Health.

Another example of service improvement using technology is the electronic prescription service, also established within Connecting for Health. The prescription is sent online, from the doctor to the pharmacy, and a text message can be sent to inform the patient when the prescription is ready for collection. In some areas of the UK, pharmacy services will deliver medicines directly to the patient.

Repeat prescriptions are automatically processed reducing the problem of the patient missing their medicines.

14.5.1
Technology to Support Patients

So far this discussion has explored the use of technology to assist health-care professionals but there are also systems available to the public. "My Health Space" is system which allows an individual to "build" their own online personal health organizer (www.healthspace.nhs.uk). In time it will be possible for the patients to access their NHS summary care record.

14.5.2
Tele Terminology

The terms telehealth, telemonitoring, telemedicine, and e-health are often used interchangeably, but there are significant differences; see Glossary.

A simpler term might be assistive technology but understanding tele terminology will help the reader to identify which type of telehealth product might be most suitable for a patient, and a potential purchaser can determine what sort of telehealth product they are shown.

The Royal College of Nursing uses the term e-health to refer to the whole scope of information and communication technology usage in health and health care (www.rcn.org.

uk/development/practice/e-health) but suggests telehealth is "the preferred overarching term, as it seems to be more inclusive and multidisciplinary in scope."[14]

14.5.3
Innovative Technology and Communication

The development in technology is vast. Simple to sophisticated products are available to meet the needs of patients and health-care professionals. Clothing that can record heart rate, sensors that can detect if a patient has fallen out of bed and generate an emergency call, monitors that can take recordings and relay the information by a standard telephone line to a health-care professional, or reminders of health appointments by text message – the explosion in technology can play a vital role in health care, not only in the future, but right now. The examples just mentioned are all available. Online social virtual worlds are a reality, and virtual wards assist student nurses to learn.

It has been suggested that even the social networking sites Facebook and Twitter could be an ideal conduit for health communication.

When put into context the potential of unexpected sources can be useful in health care. The Met Office, which provides daily weather forecasts on the radio and television in the UK, has developed a health weather alert. Weather alerts in the form of an automated telephone message inform susceptible patients of forthcoming weather likely to have an impact on their health. The aim is to encourage the patient to take a more active approach to keeping well before the arrival of weather likely to affect their health. For example, patients with COPD can receive a cold weather alert (www.metoffice.gov.uk/coldweatheralert). This service may be extended in the near future to patients with asthma to alert them of a high pollen count, and to sufferers of arthritis to alert them of cold wet weather ahead.

Some telehealth devices combine aspects of telehealth, by having a monitoring facility and the ability to ask the patient questions and provide knowledge about health conditions and further sources of support.

One example of this type of technology sends a short series of questions to the patient each day. The patient's responses travel via a standard telephone line to a secure server which can be accessed by the nurse doctor or other health-care providers. Responses are given a risk rating indicated by a yellow, green, or red flag. A red flag indicates findings that are out of the norm, prompting the need for appropriate medical or nursing action. Over time, the aim is to change the patient's behavior so that they become better self-carers and their condition becomes more stable (www.healthheronetwork).

NHS Direct (www.nhs.uk) offers a 24 hour call service and among its many activities offers support for patients with long-term conditions which may reduce the incidence of the patient calling for an emergency ambulance to hospital.

14.5.4
Understanding Technology

Technology surrounds daily life. Cash machines, digital television and cameras, and the mobile telephone are common, but telehealth equipment and computer systems are not yet integrated into the NHS across the UK.

Technology presents health-care professionals with the need to learn. A course of study in health informatics will be a useful tool, and it is suggested that this type of course is made available in the nursing and health division of universities. Currently, health informatics programs appear to be housed within the technology division and focus purely on the technology itself. A way forward would be for health care professionals and technology professionals to collaborate to design a program specifically for are professionals. To reflect the possibilities current technology offers, this could be delivered using the approach of blended learning, practical experience in the workplace, supported with a university level accredited online e-learning program.

14.6
Regulation

Telehealth is a relatively new field and as such developers within the industry are not regulated. Recently, however, the Telecare Services Association (www.telecare.org.uk), the representative body for the telecare industry in the UK, has developed a code of practice which can only enhance the standing of the industry.

"Make IT Safe"[15] is a new publication from the RCN (www.rcn.org.uk_assets) containing guidance for nursing staff using computers and IT to ensure confidentiality and safe practice.

14.7
Conclusion

IT, communication technology, and telehealth are here to stay. National IT programs support these and a range of products is available in the market place. Policies and recommendations support the use of technology to improve care to those most in need. Education and trainning programs are needed, along with regulation within the telehealth industry, to ensure that high standards of care and safe practice are achieved to meet Lord Darzi's recommendations to provide the patient with high-quality, safe, and efficient care.

14.8
Summary

The important points explored and discussed in this chapter are the following:

- Individual countries in the UK have developed some strategies to meet the challenges in providing health and social care in relation to the future health needs of their country. Government policies are driving the changes forward.
- Role of the community matron in England is perceived to be vital to the ongoing care of patients in the community in that country. The educational development of the community matron is discussed.

- Use of technology in the NHS is discussed and other examples given to demonstrate how technological solutions are improving services for patients.
- The manner in which the workforce needs to be prepared is discussed. Changes in the way nurses, doctors, and allied health professionals work cannot be overlooked.
- Nurses need to develop further skills to equip them for competent use and application of technology to support patients.

Glossary

e-health – The whole scope of information and communication technology usage in health and health care.

Telecare triage – The use of technology to aid patient assessment diagnosis and interpretation of information, for example, in the form of X-rays or scans. Tele-education involves the use of communications technology for the purpose of learning and can be used by patients or health professionals.

Telemedicine – The delivery of medical services at a distance such as consultation with a clinician between the patient's home and the doctor's surgery or even a facility in a different part of the country, using visual technology such as a web cam placed in the patient's home and a computer screen in the doctor' surgery or hospital.

Telemonitoring – Associated with telehomecare and telesupport and is the process of using monitoring equipment placed in the patient's home that can record information such as blood pressure or weight measurement which is relayed via a standard telephone line to the doctor, nurse, or other health-care professional.

References

1. Crosbie B. Discharge planning. *Br J Community Nurs.* 1999;4(1557):320.
2. Department of Health. *Achieving Timely Simple Discharge from Hospital: A Toolkit for the Multidisciplinary Team.* London: DH; 2004.
3. Department of Health. *Delivering the NHS Improvement Plan – The Workforce Contribution.* London: DH; 2004.
4. Department of Health. *Supporting People with Long Term Conditions: An NHS and Social Care Model to Support Local Innovation and Integration.* London: DH; 2005.
5. Department of Health. *Caring for People with Long-Term Conditions: An Education Framework for Community Matrons and Case Managers.* London: DH; 2006.
6. Department of Health. *Modernising Nursing Careers – Setting the Direction.* London: DH; 2006.
7. Department of Health. *A High Quality Workforce.* London: DH; 2008.
8. Department of Health. *High Quality Care for All.* London: DH; 2008.
9. Department of Health. *Modernising Allied Health Professionals (AHP) Careers: A Competence Based Career Framework.* London: DH; 2008.
10. Department of Health. *NHS Constitution for England.* London: DH; 2009.

11. Evercare. Implementing the Evercare programme: interim report; 2004. www.natpact.nhs.uk/186.php.
12. Moussavi S, Chatterji S, Verdes E, et al. Depression, chronic disease and decrements in health: results from the world health surveys. *Lancet.* 2008;370(9590):851-858.
13. Royal College of Nursing. *Agenda for Change.* London: RCN; 2004.
14. Royal College of Nursing. *Putting Information at the Heart of Nursing Care.* London: RCN; 2006.
15. Royal College of Nursing. *Make IT Safe.* London: RCN; 2009.
16. Sutherland K, Coyle D. *Quality in Healthcare in England, Wales, Scotland, Northern Ireland: An Intra UK Chart Book.* Scotland: The Health Foundation; 2009.
17. The Scottish Government. Partnership for care; 2003.
18. The Scottish Government. Better health better care: action plan; 2007.
19. Welsh Assembly Government. Designed for Life – Creating World Class Health and Social Care for Wales in the 21st Century, a Strategy for Health and Social Care in Wales; 2005.
20. Designed for Life – Creating World Class Health and Social Care for Wales in the 21st Century, a Strategy for Health and Social Care in Wales; 2005. Welsh Assembly Government.

Telenursing in New Zealand

15

Ian St George and Janet Harp

Abbreviations

ED   Emergency Department
GP   General Practitioner
NHS   National Health Service

Primary care nurses have given advice and assessed the severity of symptoms by telephone since telephones were introduced and in 1993 Tisdale[29] reported a pilot service in four small New Zealand centers, with nurses answering telephone health queries using simple diagnostic software and health databases. While it was not popular enough to warrant continuing, Tisdale wrote that this type of service "could be a valuable addition to health care services if extended nation-wide."

15.1
Drivers

By 2000, a number of drivers combined to suggest that a coordinated and professional approach to telenursing should be introduced in New Zealand.

- Nurses in general medical practices and emergency departments have traditionally triaged calls and are effective in reducing doctor's workload.[6] Currently available telephone advice was variable in quality: Aitken and her colleagues had found in 1995 that the advice given by phone from 30 New Zealand emergency departments and 20 accident and emergency clinics was inadequate from 16 of the 36 institutions that would even give advice. They used the case of a 5-week-old infant with fever. Ten clinics did not even ask the age, 27 did not ask the temperature, and 35 did not ask about the administration of paracetamol. In one clinic, the call was handled by a medical student.

I. St George (✉)
Medibank Health Solutions NZ Ltd, P.O. Box 10-643, Wellington, New Zealand
e-mail: ian.stgeorge@medibankhealth.co.nz

S. Kumar and H. Snooks (eds.), *Telenursing*, Health Informatics,
DOI: 10.1007/978-0-85729-529-3_15, © Springer-Verlag London Limited 2011

In ten clinics, the person answering was not identified; in two it was a receptionist.[1] Similar findings had been reported from Australia and the United States.

- Demand management projects were working well elsewhere: people could be helped to use health services more astutely. Such education could be seen as an empowerment helping people take better control of their health by seeking care wisely. Its critics accused demand management of trying to reduce cost at the expense of safety: its proponents claimed it could reduce cost while enhancing safety and quality of care: by educating the patient to seek care at the right place and at the right time.

- Advances in information technology allowed the creation of sophisticated computer software for triaging symptoms and keeping a clinical record and audit trail.

- Advances in telephony now allowed telephone access to a single call center for large populations; it was already commonplace for applications such as banking, travel, and computer assistance, and could now be employed for health advice. Health call center services in other countries ranged from primary triage to determine the level and timing of care needed, to the management of chronic illness.

- Other primary care services – general medical practices and emergency departments – were being overused by people presenting with minor, self-limiting, or nonurgent problems.

- On the other hand, certain populations appeared to perceive barriers to existing primary care services, especially for reporting current symptoms, and thus either underused them or presented only when their illness had deteriorated: in New Zealand these included Māori, the elderly and the socioeconomically deprived.

- Telenursing triage services were being used or trialed in other countries – NHS Direct in England, and various private programs in the United States. The safety and effectiveness of telephone triage by nurses had been demonstrated in Britain.[11,23] In the United States, over 90% of callers were satisfied with a nurse triage service,[19] the service was cost-effective[18,21] and adherence to advice was similar to that for telephone-based physician recommendations.[17]

Thus, technological advances combined with a need for demand management permitted the introduction of a new service to address social needs. That new service was funded by the New Zealand Government's Ministry of Health, which contracted McKesson New Zealand (now Medibank Health Solutions) to provide "Healthline."

Since then newer telenursing projects – for primary care triage, well child and parenting advice, advice and information on immunization, mental health assessment and support, and disease management – have been introduced, but none has been as large, or as thoroughly evaluated, as Healthline.

15.2
Healthline

The initial aims in introducing the service were thus related to equity, safety, consistency, and economy. A free telephone advice line would be accessible to all, especially to those for whom cost and rural remoteness posed barriers to existing primary care services. It would provide consistent evidence-based advice. Furthermore, it would manage demand so people who were uncertain what level of care they should seek would be directed to the right place, and at the right time; they would be supported in coping with their minor illnesses at home, freeing emergency departments, and general practices for more serious work.[25]

Healthline began in 2000 in four pilot areas of New Zealand: Gisborne and east coast North Island (very rural, high Māori population), Northland (urban and rural, high Māori population), Westland (rural and remote), and Canterbury (urban and rural). Evaluation of the results would determine whether the service was extended nationwide. Telenurses could take calls from people seeking advice about any health matter, about providers in their region, or about current symptoms.

Decision support software in the form of symptom-based guidelines supported Healthline's telenurses in triaging current symptoms. The guidelines were designed to help the nurse rule out important conditions (however rare) and stop at the condition that could not be excluded; they thus set the level and timing of the intervention. They could triage patients safely to appropriate care, while at the same time providing comprehensive automated call documentation and reporting for analysis, risk management, and quality improvement.

Callers could telephone a free number 24 h a day, 7 days a week. The nurse created a caller chart, identified the caller region, recorded the clinical complaint, selected and traversed the appropriate guideline, reached a triage outcome or endpoint, searched for an appropriate provider or offered self-care advice, and referred if necessary.

Endpoints of the call were as follows:

- *Emergency*: immediate ambulance call-out and transfer required.
- *Urgent care*: caller advised to seek care via emergency department or general practitioner within 2–24 h.
- *Speak to provider*: caller advised to speak to their general practitioner or other provider within time specified (2–24 h).
- *Appointment*: caller advised to seek nonurgent care from their general practitioner during regular hours; 3-day or 2-week timeframe specified.
- *Self-care*: caller advised on self-care measures. Follow-up call offered.

Telenursing standards were developed and approved by the Nursing Council, the regulatory authority for nursing in New Zealand.

After an independent evaluation had judged the pilot a success, Healthline became a national program in 2005. It remains a free, 24 × 7 program, in which nurses give advice supported by clinical software, and their activities are recorded and analyzed by sophisticated information technology.

15.3
The Population

New Zealand is a south Pacific island nation of four million people, 68% of whom are of European ethnic origin, 15% indigenous Māori, and the remainder largely Pacific island people and people of Asian origin.[16]

Healthline can take 324,000 calls a year: in the quarter April–June 2010 telenurses handled 87,283 calls, 67% of them outside business hours. Surveys repeatedly find 99.5% consumer satisfaction.[9] About a third of Healthline calls are at night, a third at weekends, and a third during business hours; 9 AM to 9 PM are the busy hours, and that trend is accentuated at weekends, thus suggesting that Healthline is used as an alternative source of primary care advice when other services are perceived to be less easily available. The busiest day ever was during the H1N1 influenza pandemic when over 4,000 calls were made.

15.4
Reaching Those in Greatest Need

15.4.1
Socioeconomic Deprivation

George expressed the concern that NHS Direct, the similar British service, may in fact be serving the needs of the "worried and well middle classes,"[7] a position supported by a survey showing lower awareness of the service among those in social classes D and E.[15] The UK House of Commons Public Accounts Committee recommended NHS Direct should act to encourage use by disadvantaged groups.[14]

Burt and coworkers[3] used postcode data to identify the address wards of callers to NHS Direct South East London over 6 months. They found that calls rose with increasing deprivation, until, at extreme levels of deprivation, they declined. Their results challenge the assumption that NHS Direct is not used in deprived areas.

Cooper and coworkers[4] similarly examined 6 months of calls to West Yorkshire and West Midlands NHS Direct sites, and found that call rates were highest in the middle of the range of deprivation; they concluded that overall demand for NHS Direct was highest in areas where deprivation is at or just above the national average. Furthermore, they found that at extreme deprivation, adult call rates were high, but those about children lower.[4]

The NZDep2006 Index of Deprivation combines nine variables from the 2006 census, which reflect eight dimensions of deprivation. It provides a deprivation score for each meshblock in New Zealand. Meshblocks are geographical units defined by Statistics New Zealand, containing a median of about 90 people.

The index ordinal scale ranges from 1 to 10, where 1 represents the areas with the least deprived scores and 10 the areas with the most: deprivation scores apply to areas rather than to individual people but have been extensively used as a proxy for socioeconomic deprivation where individual scores are not available.

We used the earlier NZ Dep2001 (from the 2001 census data) to examine deprivation levels of people calling Healthline in 2005.[28] The results are shown in Fig. 15.1, which replicates Burt's London results: the highest users of Healthline were people from regions with high – but not the highest – deprivation scores. The result was encouraging: healthcare need is related to socioeconomic status, and socioeconomic status matches deprivation index.

Fig. 15.1 Distribution of calls to Healthline by deprivation decile, compared with distribution of New Zealand population

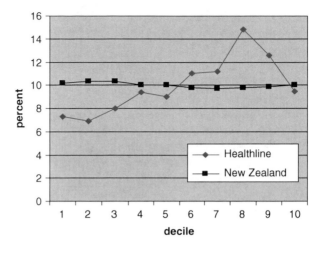

Fig. 15.2 Percent of cell phone callers ($n = 132$) in each NZDep06 decile of deprivation, compared with percent of landline callers ($n = 873$) in each decile

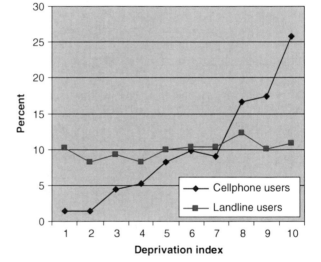

Cell phone use has increased so that by 2009 20% of calls were made by cell phone (cell phone calls to Healthline are cost-free to the caller). People in the regions with the highest deprivation scores were most likely to call by cell phone (probably reflecting the availability of prepaid cell phone plans; Fig. 15.2, unpublished data).

15.4.2
Māori

The Ministry of Health's objective in establishing the service was to increase access to health advice and services by population groups, which currently had poor access or utilization. Māori were identified as one of those populations.

Māori are overrepresented in the most socioeconomically deprived areas (more than half of all Māori live in areas represented by the three most deprived deciles) – what Reid and others called a "disparity gap."[22] As they pointed out, within disparities there is always an "outcome gap" – that is, even allowing for deprivation, the health outcomes of Māori are different from those of non-Māori.

No study of access to telephone triage by indigenous people had been published. The equivalent British system, NHS Direct, was underused by ethnic minorities, people older than 65 years and disadvantaged groups in comparison with the general population, despite the acknowledgment these groups had "as much need as others and perhaps an even greater one."[13]

Davis found that rates of general practitioner contact for Māori were slightly lower than those for non-Māori patients, so there is a limited correspondence between ethnic patterns of general practitioner usage and health need (as measured by mortality levels and rates of public hospital discharge). He concluded, "The near equivalence in ethnic rates of general practitioner contact revealed in this study contrasts strikingly both with the level of hospitalisation for Māori, which is nearly double that of nonmāori, and with the difference in mortality rates (30% higher for Māori). Attention devoted to improving access to general practitioner services among Māori may be necessary if important areas of ill health and hospital resource use are to be addressed effectively."[5]

From the outset Healthline engaged with Māori and utilized the services of a Māori advisor. Communication with Māori initially included consultation with local Māori health providers and local tribes (iwi). This was followed by targeted information and regular interviews by the Māori advisor and site director on community/iwi radio and for Māori publications. National Māori media such as *Te Karere*, *Mana News*, *Mana Tangata*, and *Whenua* were utilized whenever relevant. Particularly in Northland, local "ambassadors" (often health professionals or community leaders) were enlisted to advise about Healthline and leave material with people they met in the course of their community visits.

We studied Māori utilization of Healthline in 2000–2002: 15.1% of callers were identified as Māori (cf. 14.6% of the population). Of Māori callers 79% were seeking symptom triage, as compared with 66% for non-Māori. Otherwise there were no important differences between the characteristics of Māori and non-Māori callers.[24]

Slightly higher than expected utilization by Māori has persisted in every period since the original study.

15.4.3
The Elderly

Published opinion is that telephone triage services are underused by older people compared with their need.

In July 2001, the Medical Care Research Unit at the University of Sheffied reported,

> … use of NHS Direct … among older adults is lower than we might expect. Although this may reflect the greater experience and knowledge of older people in dealing with health and health care, it is possible that it represents an increasing marginalisation of older people from accessing services through 'new technologies' such as the telephone, the web, email or digital TV.[12]

Fig. 15.3 Ratio of the distribution of patient-initiated GP encounters ("WaiMedCa" study) to population, and ratio of the distribution of Healthline callers to population, by age group

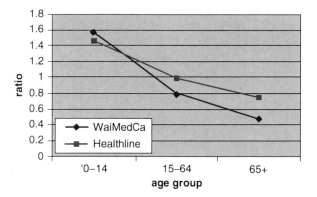

The Report in January 2002 of the UK Comptroller and Auditor General suggested NHS Direct should "target effort at both a national and local level to reach those groups with lower than average awareness and/or usage of NHS Direct" – including older people.[15]

The House of Commons Committee of Public Accounts noted that some groups, including people older than 65 years, were either less aware of NHS Direct or used it less, but had an equal or greater need of the service as those who did use it.[14]

A group of medical students questioned patients in London general practice waiting rooms and found that, even among older people who were aware of the service, actual use was lower than among younger people. Whereas younger people who had not used the service said that they had not needed to, older people (as might be expected of this sample) said that they would rather see their general practitioner.[30]

Such observations are at variance with the high use of other primary care services by the elderly – though that high use is largely because of chronic illness surveillance, rather than for advice on managing acute symptoms, which is the work of telenursing triage.

We studied the use of Healthline between 2000 and 2003 by those older than 65 years.[27] In Fig. 15.3, follow-up encounters initiated by general medical practitioners have been extracted from general practice study data, and the figure shows the ratios of the distribution of Healthline callers by age group to the population in that age group, compared with the ratio of the distribution of *patient-initiated* general practitioner encounters by age group to their population by age group (figures from McAvoy et al.[10]). There is no difference.

15.4.4
Summary

Healthline has succeeded in reaching those in greatest need: use by lower socioeconomic groups is consistently higher than that by higher socioeconomic groups, use by Māori is consistently higher than that by other ethnic groups, and use by the aged is similar to their patient-initiated consultation rate in general medical practice.

15.5
Managing Demand

Callers are asked, "What would you have done if Healthline had not been available?" Figure 15.4 shows the triage endpoints for those whose intention had been to call 111 (the emergency number in New Zealand), go to the emergency department, call their general practitioner urgently, seek nonurgent care, or self-manage. For those who had intended to call 111, only 8% needed to do so, 31% needed urgent medical care at ED or from their GP, 23% needed nonurgent care and 32% could self-manage with some education. At the other end of the scale, of those who intended self-care, a few did need advice to seek higher levels of care after triage.

In the October–December 2008 quarter, of the 32,605 callers who would have sought help elsewhere, 68% were directed to a different level of care than they would have sought if Healthline had not been available.

Thus, significant numbers of people with symptoms were unable to judge their urgency or their severity, with the result that they would have sought care inappropriately. Many stated that they would have sought a higher level of care than was judged necessary after triage; a few stated that they would have managed their symptom with a low level of care, when the triage endpoint suggested urgency. In general, however, there was a shift after triage to a lower level of care than had been intended before the call.

We studied an urban emergency department and a large rural general practice to see what, if any, effect diverting calls to Healthline would have. The intervention resulted in lower workload for emergency department nursing staff charged with answering advice calls[8] (Fig. 15.5) and lower workload for the duty doctor in the rural practice.[26] We see a major role for Healthline in managing after-hours primary care demand.

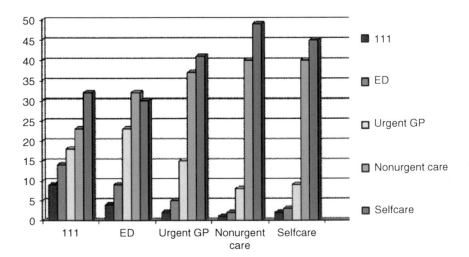

Fig. 15.4 Level of care intentions and endpoints

Fig. 15.5 Emergency department patient advice call volume

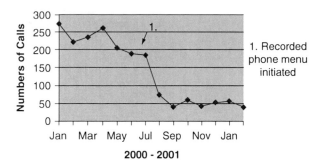

1. Recorded phone menu initiated

15.6
What Else Can a National Health Call Center Do?

15.6.1
Syndromic Surveillance

A triage line can be used for a national public health system of symptom surveillance. The term "syndromic surveillance" has been used for such activities.

Public health surveillance serves many functions, but one important task is outbreak detection – identifying a rise in frequency of disease above the background pattern. Currently, outbreaks are recognized from accumulated reports of notifiable diseases, via voluntary reporting by sentinel practices and laboratories, or by alert clinicians bringing clusters of diseases to attention.

Now the threats of bioterrorism and pandemic influenza, and the advent of a national telephone triage service, with its ready availability of electronic data, have triggered new surveillance systems to detect outbreaks earlier. These systems detect unusual geographic or temporal clustering of symptoms, and thus provide an early alert that may indicate an outbreak.

Health Ministry staff collect symptomatic data for influenza-like illnesses from Healthline data, and significant statistical excesses ("exceedances") are automatically highlighted and assessed. The team considers the age distribution, seasonal baselines, previous exceedances, and current known community levels of disease. A geocoding system can then be used to map the call addresses to check locality clustering. If concerns persist, local health protection teams are alerted.

Since 2007, Healthline data have been used alongside sentinel practice data to map influenza epidemiology in New Zealand.

Figure 15.6 traces the calls for advice about influenza-like illness associated with the 2009 H1N1 influenza pandemic. An initial small peak in late April of well callers seeking advice about contacts during the "containment" phase was followed in June and July by a massive increase in the number of symptomatic callers: special arrangements were required to try to manage the demand. A "second wave" followed in early August 2010.

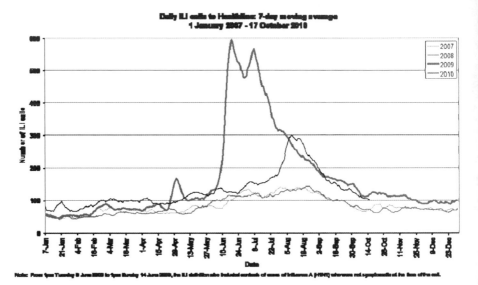

Fig. 15.6 Daily calls for influenza-like illness to Healthline: 7-day moving average (January 1, 2007–October 17, 2010)

15.6.2
Mental Health Line

The Mental Health Line is a telephone-based service, available 24 h a day, 7 days a week. Calls are diverted to the line from existing District Health Board mental health service telephone numbers.

The service assesses a service user's mental health-care needs and risk, based on the reported symptoms; uses a standardized, computerized risk assessment tool; routes them to an appropriate level and timing of mental health service; identifies the time within which that should happen; and provides mental health information and general support.

It aims to improve access to information about mental illness, improve access to services, increase the opportunity for early intervention, provide seamless service delivery, ensure appropriate referral, and enhance quality, efficiency, and effectiveness of the delivery of mental health services by reducing unnecessary demand and directing consumers to the most appropriate mental health-care services first time.

15.6.3
Chronic Disease Management

Disease management programs for chronically sick people are proliferating elsewhere, and are being piloted in New Zealand, because chronic illness accounts for most health expenditure. "The personal and economic burden of a rapidly ageing population with its inherent challenge on how better to manage chronic disease represents the next global crisis" is the slogan repeated in every issue of *DM World e-Report*.

General practitioners will not be able to manage chronic illness without help: "If the typical family physician were to follow current guidelines for the 10 most common chronic diseases, the amount of time required would exceed the time we currently have for direct patient care overall, leaving *no* time for acute illnesses or delivery of preventive services."[20]

Clearly, a cooperative approach between primary medical services and telenursing will have a place in chronic disease management in New Zealand.

15.6.4
Other Applications

Bentley listed the activities of the McKesson Asia Pacific health call center in Perth, and in doing so listed some of the possibilities for future telenursing in New Zealand[2]: *HealthDirect* triage and advice, *HealthInfo* information and health policy, *SouthWest24* mental health services, *Residential Care Line*, *Sexual Assault Referral Centre Crisis Line*, *Drug Cautioning Line*, *Health Incident Lines* (public health emergency lines as required, e.g., SARS line), and *PEP* (postexposure prophylaxis for HIV). Programs being piloted were *Secondary triage for the St John Ambulance*, *Chest pain program* for insured patients, *Outpatient bookings* (an appointment, reminder, and tracking system), and *Surgical patient follow up*. Medibank Health Sydney centre runs the mental health service *Greater Murray Access Line*, as well as a gambling line, and chronic disease management.

There will be many unforeseen possibilities to add to that list: the future of telenursing appears very promising in New Zealand.

15.7
Summary

- By 2000, a number of drivers combined to suggest that a coordinated and professional approach to telenursing should be introduced in New Zealand.
- Technological advances combined with a need for demand management resulted in a new service to address social needs – "Healthline."
- Healthline became a national program in 2005. It remains a free, 24 × 7 program, in which nurses give advice supported by clinical software.
- Healthline has succeeded in reaching those in greatest need: use by lower socioeconomic groups higher than by higher socioeconomic groups, use by Māori higher than use by other ethnic groups, and use by the aged is similar to their patient-initiated consultation rate in general medical practice.
- Since 2007, Healthline data have been used alongside sentinel practice data to map influenza epidemiology in New Zealand.
- The Mental Health Line is a telephone-based service, available 24 × 7, which assesses a service user's mental health-care needs and risk, using a standardized, computerized risk assessment tool, and provides mental health information and general support.
- A cooperative approach between primary medical services and telenursing will have a place in chronic disease management in New Zealand.

References

1. Aitken ME, Carey MJ, Kool B. Telephone advice about an infant given by after-hours clinics and emergency departments. *N Z Med J*. 1995;108(1005):315-317.
2. Bentley PJ, Turner VF, Hodgson SA, et al. A central role for the health call centre. *Aust Health Rev*. 2005;29:435-438.
3. Burt J, Hooper R, Jessopp L. The relationship between use of NHS Direct and deprivation in southeast London: an ecological analysis. *J Public Health Med*. 2003;25(2):174-176.
4. Cooper D, Arnold E, Hollyoak V, et al. The effect of deprivation, age and sex on NHS Direct call rates. *Br J Gen Pract*. 2005;55:287-291.
5. Davis P, Lay-Yee R, Sinclair O, et al. Maori/non-Maori patterns of contact, expressed morbidity and resource use in general practice: data from the Waikato Medical Care Survey 1991–2. *N Z Med J*. 1997;110:390-392.
6. Gallagher M, Huddart T, Henderson B. Telephone triage of acute illness by a practice nurse in general practice: outcomes of care. *Br J Gen Pract*. 1998;48(429):1141-1146.
7. George S. NHS Direct audited. *Br Med J*. 2002;324:558-559.
8. Graber DJ, O'Donovan P, Ardagh MW, et al. A telephone advice line does not decrease the number of presentations to Christchurch Emergency Department, but does decrease the number of phone callers seeking advice. *N Z Med J*. 2003;116(1177):495-501.
9. Healthline Quarterly Report to New Zealand Ministry of Health, unpublished; 41 (April–June 2010).
10. McAvoy B, Davis P, Raymont A, et al. The Waikato Medical Care (WaiMedCa) Survey 1991–1992. *N Z Med J*. 1994;107(Suppl 2):387-433.
11. Munro J, Nicholl JP, O'Cathain A, et al. *Evaluation of NHS Direct First Wave Sites: First Interim Report to the Department of Health*. Sheffield: Medical Care Research Unit; 1998.
12. Munro J, Nicholl J, O'Cathain A, et al. *Evaluation of NHS Direct First Wave Sites: Final Report of the Phase 1 Research*. University of Sheffield: Medical Care Research Unit; 2001: 71-72.
13. National Audit Office, United Kingdom. Report on NHS Direct; 2002. www.nao.gov.uk Accessed January 27, 2009.
14. NHS Direct in England. *House of Commons Committee of Public Accounts, HC610*. London: The Stationery Office; 2000.
15. NHS Direct in England. *Report of the Comptroller and Auditor General*. England: National Audit Office; 2002:4.
16. NZ Government Statistics Department. Census; 2006. http://www.stats.govt.nz/NR/rdonlyres/E62BDFE7-FE39-4730-B1BD-563CC3D414C0/35756/QuickStatsPopulationandDwellings1.xls. Accessed January 27, 2009.
17. O'Connell JM, Towles W, Yin M, et al. Patient adherence to telephone-based nurse triage recommendations. *Med Decis Mak*. 2000;22(4):309-317.
18. O'Connell JM, Johnson DA, Stallmeyer J, et al. A satisfaction and cost-effectiveness study of a nursing triage service. *Am J Manag Care*. 2001;7(2):159-169.
19. O'Connell JM, Stanley JL, Malakar L. Satisfaction and patient outcomes of a telephone-based nurse triage service. *Manag Care*. 2001;10:55-65.
20. Ostbye T, Yarnall KSH, Drause KM, et al. Is there time for management of patients with chronic diseases in primary care? *Ann Fam Med*. 2005;3:209-214.
21. Plocher DW, Parrott M, O'Connell JM. A cost-benefit study of a telephone-based nurse triage service; 2000. Unpublished manuscript.
22. Reid P, Robson B, Jones CP. Disparities in health: common myths and uncommon truths. *Pac Health Dialog*. 2000;7(1):38-47.

23. South Wiltshire Out-of-hours Project Group (SWOOP). Nurse telephone triage in out of hours primary care: a pilot study. *Br Med J.* 1997;314:198-199.
24. St George IM, Branney M, Horo-Gregory W, et al. Maori callers to a telephone triage service. *NZ Fam Phys.* 2003;30:261-263.
25. St George IM, Cullen M, Branney M. A primary care demand management pilot in New Zealand: telephone triage using symptom-based algorithms. *Asia Pac Fam Med.* 2003;2:153-156.
26. St George IM, Cullen M, Branney M, et al. Telephone triage reduces out-of-hours work for country doctors. *NZ Fam Phys.* 2003;30:95-99.
27. St George IM, Cullen M, Branney M. How well does telephone triage meet the needs of older people? *NZ Fam Phys.* 2005;32:94-97.
28. St George IM, Cullen MJ, Branney M. The deprivation profile and ethnicity of Healthline callers. *NZ Fam Phys.* 2006;33(6):386-389.
29. Tisdale G. The results of a telephone health advice and information service February–March 1993. *N Z Med J.* 1994;107(975):128-129.
30. Theivendra A, Sood V, Vasireddy A, et al. Men and older people are less likely to use NHS Direct. *Br Med J.* 2003;326:710.

Telenursing in the United States

16

Janet L. Grady

Abbreviations

ATA	American Telemedicine Association
CCHT	Care Coordination/Home Telehealth
NTAI	Nursing Telehealth Applications Initiative
VA	Veterans' Administration

16.1
Telenursing Defined

Ask an average citizen what nurses do and where and how they do it. Shaped by the popular media, the answer is likely to describe nurses dressed in white uniforms scurrying around a central station in a hospital unit or emergency department, performing treatments or administering medications to their patients lying in bed in the surrounding rooms. While this scenario still exists in many traditional health-care settings, nurses are also practicing in a variety of less traditional arenas, one of which involves telehealth nursing, or telenursing.

Telenursing has been defined by Milholland[2] as the removal of time and distance barriers for the delivery of health-care services or related health-care activities, and by Skiba and Barton[3] as the use of telecommunications technology in nursing to enhance patient care. Telenursing involves the use of various technologies to transmit data, voice, and video communication signals. It can include the use of telephones, computers, videophones, and other more sophisticated devices that enable nurses to practice nursing in nontraditional ways. One example of a nontraditional approach to the delivery of nursing care is when the patient and the nurse providing care to that patient are not in the same physical location. Another example is when the nurse and patient are together but located

J.L. Grady
Nursing Program at UPJ,
University of Pittsburgh at Johnstown, 141 Biddle Hall, Johnstown, PA 15904, USA
e-mail: jgrady@pitt.edu

S. Kumar and H. Snooks (eds.), *Telenursing*, Health Informatics,
DOI: 10.1007/978-0-85729-529-3_16, © Springer-Verlag London Limited 2011

at a distance from another provider, such as a physician or other specialist, needed to provide care or consultation to the patient. From these examples, one might glean that telenursing is useful in providing not only direct patient care, but also care management and coordination.

16.2
What Telenurses Do

Nurses who deliver care in nontraditional settings or who use nontraditional approaches to deliver care are first and foremost practicing nursing. The Telehealth Nursing Special Interest group of the American Telemedicine Association (ATA) has developed a white paper to help explain the field of telehealth nursing and various telehealth applications used by telenurses. The white paper, which can be accessed from the ATA website, is useful in providing a framework for the development of guidelines and standards for telenursing practice. Telehealth nursing leaders who authored the white paper explain that "the body of nursing knowledge and competencies remain constant; it is merely the medium of delivery that is different from traditional nursing care." In other words, all clinical, legal, and ethical guidelines for traditional nursing practice apply equally to nontraditional approaches such as telenursing. Telenurses are still nurses, but the use of various technologies enables them to extend the reach of nursing care to patients who might not otherwise have access, or whose access would be severely restricted if limited to traditional approaches only.

16.3
Telenurses and Their Roles – Sharon Daley

One nurse who has been able to extend the reach of care through telenursing is Sharon Daley, who lives on an island off the coast of Maine. For the past 9 years, Sharon has worked for the Maine Seacoast Mission, which provides needed care for island inhabitants. Although the mission has a long history of serving the islands, the use of telenursing is a more recent addition, beginning with the outfitting of a patient examination room on a 72-ft boat. Sharon regularly places posters on each island to announce when she will be there and which providers will be available on the mainland via telehealth technology. On the boat, Sharon functions as the telepresenter, assisting the provider on the mainland to obtain health assessments and other information from the patient. In addition to primary care physicians, Sharon works with other specialists from areas ranging from diabetes care and behavioral health to child psychiatry.

Sharon's broad experience in nursing enables her to identify articulated as well as less obvious needs of the island inhabitants. For example, Sharon notes that patients in some cases complained of physical symptoms but really did not suffer from any physical disease. While the patients may have had difficulty articulating exactly what they needed,

Sharon's nursing judgment told her that counseling may be in order. Once patients were connected to appropriate counseling resources, Sharon noticed a decrease in physical complaints. Without telehealth services, island inhabitants would be faced with the expensive and inconvenient alternative of taking several days off work to seek care on the mainland. In many cases, the chosen alternative might be to go without the needed care.

In essence, Sharon serves as a bridge to the island communities and has a sense of connection to the people who live and work there. Based on a trusting nurse–patient relationship, Sharon is able to provide a multitude of services from a children's dental program to alcoholics anonymous meetings, all through telehealth technology. "If there is a need, I try to figure out how to meet that need," states Sharon, who has also brought school nurse services, respiratory care, and medication information sessions to island inhabitants. Still, she sees unmet needs to be addressed. In the future, she would like to be able to offer speech therapy for children and additional health-care education to emergency medical personnel, teachers, and park rangers on the island. As one registered nurse leveraging telehealth technology, Sharon continues to have a huge positive impact on the health and wellness of many island inhabitants served by the Maine Seacoast Mission.

16.4
Telenurses and Their Roles – Cindy Gordon and Kathy Duckett

Cindy Gordon and Kathy Duckett have each been managing their respective telehealth programs for the past 4 years. Both were instrumental in the planning and implementation of their programs, Cindy for the Rochester Health System in Rochester, New York, and Kathy with Partners Home Care in Boston, Massachusetts. Both are excellent examples of nursing commitment, innovation, and telenursing leadership.

The program for which Cindy Gordon is Telemedicine Manager was originally established to make health care accessible in the rural setting and to provide a telehealth outpatient specialty clinic with services including cardiology, urology, radiation oncology, pulmonology, and reconstructive breast surgery, among others. The idea for a telehealth clinic grew from a vision to reach out to the many rural citizens of the Rochester Health System with poor access to health care. With circumstances similar to patients living in the islands off the coast of Maine, rural New York residents would often go without care rather than travel into the city to obtain it.

At present, the Rochester program is providing 10–15 medical consultations each week, including inpatient, outpatient, and nursing home consults. Telehealth is built into the strategic plan of the health system. According to Cindy, outpatients are now obtaining access to health care much sooner, with the need for transportation and associated expense and inconvenience eliminated. Telenurses can facilitate health assessment by providing physical examination data to providers located at a distance from the patient (see Fig. 16.1). Cindy also notes that patients are highly satisfied with the telehealth service, and that they are quick to overcome the feeling of not being in the same physical location as their provider. Sophisticated telecommunications technology enables telenurses to extend the reach of nursing care, thus leading to greater patient satisfaction (see Fig. 16.2).

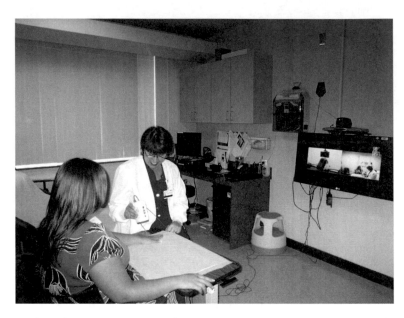

Fig. 16.1 Using a dermoscopy camera to take and transmit photos of a patient's skin condition to a remote provider

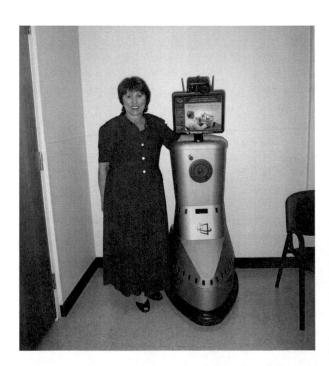

Fig. 16.2 Mobile video telecommunications equipment assists telenurses to care for patients at a distance

While the range of services provided by the Rochester telehealth program is wide, Cindy sees a huge opportunity to use the technology to manage chronic patients in the home environment, with providers either seeing patients individually in their homes or with patients going to a nearby rural clinic to be managed at a distance in a group setting. As with Sharon Daley, Cindy Gordon sees a need for additional services for children including telepsychiatry. Cindy believes that increasing public awareness about the availability and effectiveness of telehealth technology will be important in promoting its acceptance as a delivery method. Wisely she states, "Once people know they can ask for it, many will demand to have it as part of their health care regime."

Like Cindy Gordon, Kathy Duckett brings years of nursing experience to her role as Director of Clinical Programs for Partners Home Care. When Kathy joined Partners Home Care, the organization was piloting the use of home telemonitoring in an effort to decrease the frequency of in-person home visits by nurses. Kathy was charged with developing a telemonitoring program that would maintain high-quality patient care and produce positive patient outcomes while effectively utilizing finite nursing resources. Results of the pilot study demonstrated that the use of home telemonitoring was associated with fewer required in-person nurse visits, good patient outcomes, and a decrease in hospitalization rate. Along with her staff, Kathy implemented the pilot study model across the home care agency. More than 125 patients currently enrolled in the Partners Home Care home telemonitoring program participate in an asynchronous monitoring process. This means that patients use telehealth devices in their homes to send data, such as blood pressure readings, weight, and other information to a telenurse in a centralized monitoring station. The nurse reviews the data and makes decisions about contacting the patient or the patient's primary care provider. Having one telenurse in the monitoring station review the data of many patients frees the nurses in the field to see more patients, or to spend additional time with those who need more complex care.

Kathy sees the home telemonitoring program as a win–win situation, in that patients are getting the care they need in an environment they want to be in, and hospital beds are saved for those patients who really need to be there. One success story Kathy tells involves a 91-year-old patient who had been frequently readmitted to the hospital for complications of heart failure. This gentleman was enrolled in the home telemonitoring program and did not require rehospitalization during his entire 117 days in the program. Once discharged, however, he was back in the hospital within several weeks. Consistent with what many telenurses believe, Kathy is convinced that this patient needed daily telemonitoring, explaining that "he needed to know that people were paying attention, which made him pay attention … it empowered him."

It is common for patients in home telemonitoring programs to describe the increased sense of control they feel due to their participation. Most say that they would recommend it to others, and many express regret that such options were unavailable to loved ones or friends with similar medical conditions. While individuals unfamiliar with the benefits of home telemonitoring might believe that patients would feel less connected to their providers, just the opposite appears to be true. In fact, patients often say that they feel even more connected than with traditional nursing care approaches, largely because they know someone is looking at them, albeit through technology, every single day. They take comfort in knowing that if something unusual is noted in the data, a telenurse will contact them immediately so that small problems can be treated before developing into more complex issues requiring hospitalization. It is easy to understand why Kathy Duckett agrees home telemonitoring will become a standard of care for chronic disease management in the not too distant future.

16.5
Telenurses and Their Roles: Rita Kobb

Although it would be impossible to describe in one chapter the full range of services provided by telenurses, no review would be complete without including the contributions of telenurses working for the US Veterans' Administration (VA). The VA's Sunshine Healthcare Network in Florida has taken a lead role in the development, implementation, and evaluation of many types of telehealth programs and has served as the model for the VA's national care coordination/home telehealth (CCHT) program. Rita Kobb is Education Program Specialist and Director of the Sunshine Training Center, and has been a telenursing champion and leader since her program's inception in 1998. Remarkably, the program has grown from serving 482 patients in 2000 to close to 50,000 nationwide in 2009. The story behind the program's success includes the pivotal role played by Rita and other nurses committed to the improvement of health-care services for their patients. As part of her leadership role, Rita has provided telehealth training and education to many registered nurses participating in the program (see Fig. 16.3).

Prior to the program's inception, a needs assessment determined that 3–4% of the patient population served by the VA was consuming about 40% of the agency's resources. A multidisciplinary group including nurses questioned what could be done differently not only to assure appropriate and high-quality care, but also to do it in the most cost-effective manner. One solution to the problem involves the VA's approach to patient care and its

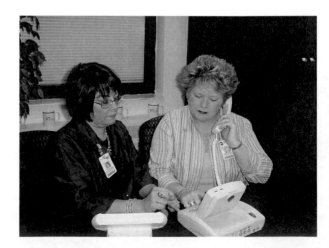

Fig. 16.3 Demonstrating the use of a videophone to connect virtually with home care patients

reimbursement. In the VA model, a system is funded with a certain amount of money to take care of a certain number of individuals, so the incentive is to keep the veteran population as healthy as possible. Money saved can be used for other areas related to patient care. According to Rita Kobb, the VA saved 23 million dollars in the first 2 years of a pilot study of its home telehealth program, and was able to shift the savings into other areas of need such as pharmacy services.

From serving on the original planning team to bringing the skills necessary for successful program implementation and evaluation, nurses are integral players in the VA's telehealth program. While the program depends on the contributions of a variety of health-care professionals, 85–90% of care coordinators, or case managers in the field, are registered nurses or nurse practitioners. Nursing presence is very evident inside the administrative structure of the program, and nurses continue to contribute in a variety of important ways in addition to patient care, such as writing practice standards and monitoring treatment protocols. Rita and her colleagues are currently planning for expanded applications of telenursing to benefit the patient population, with one example being hospice care in the home using telehealth technology. The idea is to combine the assessment, communication, and clinical skills of a nurse with the spiritual focus and unique skills of a chaplain to create a best-practice dyad to meet all of the patient's needs with the least intrusion and in the most timely way possible. Telehealth applications such as messaging devices and videophones can be used to provide spiritual care and enhance the overall quality of nursing care services. Creative telenursing approaches have not only decreased emergency room visits and conserved resources, but have also improved quality of life and decreased anxiety for hospice patients and their families.

16.6
Telenursing Role Survey

The stories of Sharon, Cindy, Kathy, and Rita illustrate only a few of the many capacities in which telenurses are practicing in the United States. However, their words echo the wisdom and commitment of telenursing colleagues throughout the country and beyond, as evidenced by results of a telenursing survey conducted several years ago. From 2003 to 2010, the author of this chapter served as Principal Investigator on a federally funded telehealth research project titled "Nursing Telehealth Applications Initiative (NTAI)." The *International Telenursing Survey*[1] was one activity within the NTAI. The survey included responses from over 700 telenurses in 30 different countries, with 68% of the respondents being from the United States. In addition to demographic information, the survey sought to explore areas including telenurses' satisfaction with their current role, perceptions about effectiveness of telehealth technology as a way to extend nursing services, and types of knowledge and skills needed by telenurses.

Ninety percent of the US sample was female, with a mean age of 48 years. Forty percent was prepared at the bachelor's degree level, 35% at the associate degree level, and 19% at the diploma level. Employers for the respondents varied widely, with the three highest percentages being hospitals, community/home care, and colleges. While close to half of the sample indicated that they had received additional formal education preparing them for advanced practice roles such as nurse practitioner or clinical nurse specialist, few had received any formal education related to telenursing roles and competencies.

Like their international colleagues, US respondents to the International Telenursing Survey expressed satisfaction with their role, based on factors including autonomy, social and professional interaction, professional status, salary, and task requirements of their job. The majority were more satisfied with their telenursing role as compared to "traditional" nursing positions they had held. Respondents predicted an increase in the need for nurses prepared to practice in telenursing roles, based on projected needs of the elderly, chronically ill, rural, underserved, and disabled populations, among others. In addition, the current challenges to our health-care system, including the need to do more with fewer resources, led respondents to view telenursing as a feasible and necessary health-care delivery strategy.

16.7
Issues and Barriers

It is clear that telenursing in the United States has made great strides over the past decade, and all indicators point to continued growth and increasing viability in the years ahead. It is equally clear, however, that there will be issues to address and barriers to overcome. Several such challenges were described by the respondents to the International Telenursing Survey and reiterated by the telenurses highlighted in this chapter. Challenges exist in the areas of education, research, policy, and acceptance.

Nursing education programs have traditionally been slow to change, even though nursing faculty recognize that changes in the practice arena must drive changes in curricula. Because nurses practicing in many different specialty areas, from pediatrics to geriatrics, and in many different settings, from home care to correctional care, will be using telenursing tools, nursing school curricula must include education to prepare students for future practice. In the cases of the telenurses described in this chapter, none received telenursing content in their basic nursing education program. In addition to on-the-job training, most did reading and exploration on their own, attended networking conferences, and utilized resources provided by various telemedicine equipment vendors and organization such as the ATA and the Association of Telehealth Service Providers. Today's nursing students would benefit from exposure to telenursing principles and practices as part of their preparation for professional practice. Graduate nurses need to be prepared not only for what they will encounter in the immediate future, but also for the possibilities that will emerge as the health-care arena changes. A vast majority of respondents to the International Telenursing Survey believed that telenursing should be part of basic nursing education and that nursing students should have clinical experiences with telehealth in addition to traditional nursing site placements. Student nurses need to understand telenursing practice, and be familiar with remote assessment equipment such as digital stethoscopes, otoscopes, wound cameras, and messaging devices that will be part of their clinical tool kit (see Fig. 16.4).

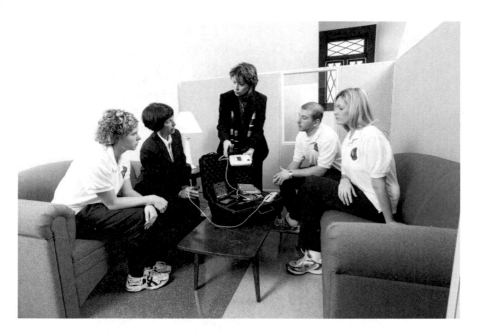

Fig. 16.4 Telenurse home – familiarizing nursing students with tools of telehealth practice for home health care

As part of her "Nursing Telehealth Applications Initiative" research project, the author of this chapter has designed and implemented experiences to expose nursing students to telehealth tools and their use in patient-care situations. One innovative adjunct to traditional nursing education strategies involved a health assessment course during which students learn techniques for in-person patient assessment as well as assessment at a distance using telehealth tools (see Fig. 16.5). For example, students first learned cardiovascular assessment for a patient they can touch; then, students learned the same cardiovascular assessment using telehealth tools such as digital stethoscopes and videoconferencing cameras to examine a patient located at a distance from the student nurse. Through the use of videoconferencing equipment connecting two practice sites, students in a health assessment class were provided opportunities to act both as telepresenter of the patient and as remote provider (see Fig. 16.5 and 16.6). Data collected following the health assessment course indicated students agreed that telehealth tools enabled accurate evaluation of patients located geographically distant from the provider. The vast majority of students saw telehealth as an effective strategy for nurses and responded that they would consider using telehealth tools in their future practice. Similar experiences should be incorporated into all nursing programs so that students are prepared for the telehealth-enhanced nursing practice arena of the future.

Future growth of telenursing will also depend in part on the quality of telenursing research to provide a foundation and framework for continued development and evaluation of telenursing applications, leading to identification and support of best, evidence-based practices. While there is a developing body of high-quality telenursing literature, there are also many small studies with little control and largely anecdotal evidence. Telenurses need

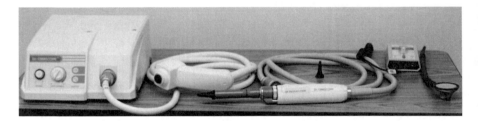

Fig. 16.5 Digital equipment to conduct long distance patient assessment

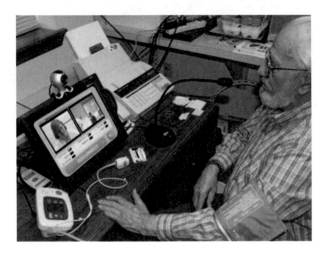

Fig. 16.6 Patient at home using telehealth equipment to communicate with nurse at a distance

to be constantly vigilant in assessing patients' needs, questioning how needs might best be met, and seeking answers to questions through nursing research. Telenurses practicing in clinical settings should partner with colleagues in the academic arena to design quality studies that will produce evidence needed to support, refine, and improve telenursing patient care.

Policy issues also present obstacles to telenursing practice, particularly in terms of nursing licensure. Nursing licensure in the United States is regulated at the level of the individual states, and in most cases, nurses must be licensed in the state where the patients they are caring for are located. While telehealth technology enables the nurse and patient to be located at physical distances from each other, licensure constraints may prohibit a nurse in one state from caring for a patient in another state (see Fig. 16.6). The National Council of State Boards of Nursing has developed the Nurse Licensure Compact, which is intended to provide state-to-state licensure portability for registered nurses. Although the compact has been supported by numerous nursing and health-care organizations, political and other issues have resulted in only 23 states thus far joining the compact.

While the full discussion of the range of policy issues is well beyond the scope of this chapter, an essential question related to telenursing is how it is reimbursed. Unlike medical consultations, there is at present no clear reimbursement mechanism for a variety of telenursing services including "virtual" home care visits, or those done using telehealth technology. It is easy to understand why health-care administrators may be hesitant to adopt and support unreimbursed telenursing services, even when they believe in the value-added services for patients as well as staff.

One area that appears to be a strength rather than a challenge is that of the telehealth technology itself. Improvements in functionality, usability, and quality of the hardware seem to be occurring on a daily basis. For example, monitoring equipment that was once cumbersome and intrusive in patients' homes can now be camouflaged as small pieces of wearable devices. Upgraded equipment with attention to ease of use has made it relatively simple for even a frail, elderly patient to participate in his own health care through tele-health technology. Staying in touch with the telenurse can be as easy as touching a button on a videophone or monitoring device. Improvements like these have led to wide accep-tance and resulting patient satisfaction. However, telehealth technology is not viewed and accepted by everyone as a legitimate and necessary tool to provide patient care. Even as patients of different ages and medical conditions have embraced the services received from their caring and committed telenurses, securing buy-in and support from other important stakeholders in the health-care environment, including some physicians, nurses, administrators, and policy makers, has been a more difficult task for telenurses.

In essence, nursing practice enhanced through the use of telehealth technology, or telenursing, has and will continue to be a positive influence on American health care. Telenursing provides one strategy to address areas of nursing resource shortages while enhancing the ability of nurses to anticipate and prevent problems, resulting in cost savings to the system and quality-of-life improvement for patients. Most importantly, telenursing has potential for increasing the reach of nursing care to populations with unmet or under-met needs. As was so eloquently stated by one telenurse in the International Telenursing Survey, "telenursing allows us to reach out our hearts through technology."

16.8
Summary

- Definitions of telenursing vary, but all refer to the use of some type of telecommunica-tions technology within the practice of nursing.
- Telenurses may use nontraditional tools and approaches to deliver patient care, but their practice is guided by traditional nursing standards.
- The "Telehealth Nursing White Paper," an educational resource developed by the Telehealth Nursing Special Interest Group of the ATA, is available on the ATA website at http://www.americantelemed.org.
- Telenurses can serve as telepresenters by assisting other distant providers, such as physi-cians, with patient examinations or consultations. Alternately, telenurses in advanced practice roles, such as nurse practitioners, can function as long-distance care providers.

- Telehealth communication technology enables telenurses to provide care to patients in rural or underserved areas, or those for whom transportation for in-person visits is difficult or impossible.
- Telenursing applications have the potential to significantly decrease costs to the healthcare system while increasing access to care and quality of life for patients.
- The "International Telenursing Role Survey," co-conducted by the chapter's author, found that telenurses are satisfied with their work and see telenursing as a way to extend the reach of their care while meeting current challenges to the health-care system.
- Nursing students need to be exposed to telenursing principles and practice in order to effectively prepare them for future nursing practice.
- Challenges related to nursing research, licensure, reimbursement, technology acceptance, and other policy issues will need to be addressed as the field of telenursing grows and evolves.

Glossary

Telehealth – A broader definition of remote health care that does not always involve clinical services. Videoconferencing transmission of still images, e-health including patient portals, remote monitoring of vital signs, continuing medical education, and nursing call centers are all considered part of telemedicine and telehealth (American Telemedicine Association).

Telehealth nursing – Used interchangeably with telenursing.

Telehealth technology – Includes various forms of telecommunications technologies such as videoconferencing. Also includes any devices that can send data over a distance, including computers, videophones, remote monitoring devices, etc.

Telemedicine – Use of medical information exchanged from one site to another via electronic communications to improve patients' health status (American Telemedicine Association).

Telepresenters – Telenurses working in the same room with patients who are participating in telehealth consultations with other health-care providers at a distance (American Telemedicine Association).

References

1. Grady JL, Schlachta-Fairchild L. Report of the 2004-2005 International Telenursing Survey. *Comput Inform Nurs*. 2007;25(5):266-272.
2. Milholland DK. Telehealth: a tool for nursing practice. *Nurs Trends Issues*. 1997;2(4):1-7, 2.
3. Skiba D, Barton A. Health-oriented communications. In: Ball MJ, Hannah KJ, Newbold SK, Douglas JV, eds. *Nursing Informatics: Where Caring and Technology Meet*. 3rd ed. New York: Springer; 2000.

Telenursing: An Audit

17

Sajeesh Kumar

17.1
Telenursing Is Advancing

Telenursing is a relatively young field; consequently, further long-term studies with regard to legal issues, cost, and safety are required before the technology can be integrated into the mainstream health-care system. Telenursing services are not going away, but the field is evolving. As with many young disciplines, telenursing seems to redefine itself on a fairly regular basis – changing to meet the demand of managing more and larger specialties. Telenursing is growing worldwide annually, due, in large part, to the approval of procedures. In addition, given better acceptance among nurses, physicians, hospitals, and patients, this growth will likely increase. It must be noted that the growth of telenursing will directly support and help the growth of nursing, because telenursing is, of course, an integral part of nursing.

17.2
Will Telenursing Replace Traditional Methods?

Telenursing promises to revolutionize nursing and speed up the health-care process. Yet, the technology requires a great deal of further development. The introduction of telenursing does not mean that nurses can abandon traditional methods. As well, the economics of telenursing must be further analyzed. Institutions must ensure that the cost of telenursing does not exceed the traditional expenses involved with nursing care.

S. Kumar
Department of Health Information Management, School of Health & Rehabilitation Sciences,
University of Pittsburgh, 6022 Forbes Tower, Pittsburgh, PA 15260, USA
e-mail: sajeeshkr@yahoo.com

S. Kumar and H. Snooks (eds.), *Telenursing*, Health Informatics,
DOI: 10.1007/978-0-85729-529-3_17, © Springer-Verlag London Limited 2011

17.3
Issues Related to Telenursing: A Brief Overview

Immediate or widespread implementation of telenursing is hindered by many factors. Issues such as reimbursement and security are still in flux.

Issues related to telenursing may also include lack of telecommunication infrastructure, affordability of programs, cost of the equipments, accuracy of the medical and nonmedical devices used, training of personnel involved, lack of guidelines and protocols, sustainability of the projects, regulations regarding sharing of information, privacy, and legal liability.

17.4
Changing Industry

What will telenursing practice look like in the coming years? To what extent and when might telenursing replace on-site nurses?

Telenursing is driven by the relative shortage of nurses – not the enabling technology.

The reality is that the local nurse has much control of this situation. The local nurse has the existing long-term community relationships and the ability to do procedures, on-site consultations, and conferences, as well as oversight in the nursing department. The biggest risk that a local nurse can take is to continue in a seriously understaffed situation. By partnering with a trusted telenursing provider, they should find that their local hospital contract is more secure than it ever has been. Anything that improves service in the local practice will, in the form of better staffing levels, make it much harder for an outsider to compete.

If hospitals and groups have an on-site option, they are going to take it. It may also contract with a telenursing company to handle overflow. Expansion may come in the bedside telenursing because that is simply when most studies are being done. Of course, physicians' turnaround expectations are getting shorter, not longer.

17.5
Money Matters

Meeting the demand is a major telenursing driver, along with economic motivation. A group already large enough to staff and share off-hour call may show an economic benefit. Besides quality nurses, a track record of adaptability might be the trait facilities, and groups need to focus on when they consider implementing telenursing technology.

Financial planning for telenursing should include the costs of telecommunication and information technology infrastructure and medical devices, as well as costs such as personnel training, monthly network access fees, maintenance, telephone bills, and other operational expenses.

Once the objectives of a program are identified, technology support personnel should be consulted, to clarify technical equipment specifications and facility requirements. Protocols and guidelines must be developed, which will provide clear direction on how to utilize telenursing most effectively. The training of nurses is especially critical in telenursing. The reliability of a program is also related to the experience with telenursing technology and the awareness of its limitations.

Many nations do not have explicit policies to pay for telenursing services. A major telenursing payment policy is crucial. Meanwhile, several telemedicine services are being integrated to regular health-care systems in the United States and the Scandinavian countries with reimbursement/payment options. Studies should be conducted to implement, monitor, evaluate, and refine the telenursing payment process. Additionally, it should be noted that telenursing licensure and indemnity laws might also need to be formulated. This issue, however, remains a cloudy region for health-care strategists and has implications for nurses and remote practitioners who practice across state or country lines.

It is observed that successful telenursing programs are often the product of careful planning, sound management, dedicated professionals and support staff, and a commitment to appropriate funding to support capital purchases and ongoing operations. It reflects a commitment to teamwork to link technical and operational complexities into a fully integrated and efficiently functioning program. Telenursing service providers, health insurance agencies, and all concerned institutions could convene to lead a workable model for telenursing service improvements. The professional communities could bring out telenursing service guidelines, which would pave the way for consensus on several difficult issues, including technical and service standardization for telenursing.

17.6
Conclusion

Health-care providers are now looking at telenursing as a model of improving, automating, and enhancing patient care. This book elaborates on many aspects of telenursing. Authors have shown telenursing to be practical, safe, and effective. Success often relates to the efficiency and effectiveness of the transfer of information and translates to improved or enhanced patient care than would otherwise be possible.

Available telenursing technology still has considerable room for improvement. However, the challenge is why, where, and how to implement which technology and at what costs. Asking the right questions will drive the technologies. A needs assessment is critical before implementing a telenursing project. Telenursing, as delineated in these pages, may appear novel but is rapidly coming into common and mundane usage through multiple applications.

Index

S. Kumar and H. Snooks (eds.), *Telenursing*, Health Informatics,
DOI: 10.1007/978-0-85729-529-3, © Springer-Verlag London Limited 2011